Quantifying Under-nutrition in Rural India

About the Author

Rekha Sharma is Associate Professor, Department of Economics, Sri Guru Gobind Singh College of Commerce, University of Delhi. She is MA, MPhil, PhD from Department of Economics, Delhi School of Economics, University of Delhi. Dr Sharma has teaching experience of 25 years in University of Delhi and has taught papers related to microeconomics and its applications and development theory & experience.

Quantifying Under-nutrition in Rural India

Rekha Sharma

ACADEMIC FOUNDATION
NEW DELHI

www.academicfoundation.org
www.academicfoundation.com

First published in 2015
by

ACADEMIC FOUNDATION
4772-73 / 23 Bharat Ram Road, (23 Ansari Road),
Darya Ganj, New Delhi - 110 002 (India).
Phones : 23245001 / 02 / 03 / 04.
Fax : +91-11-23245005.
E-mail : books@academicfoundation.com
www.academicfoundation.org
www.academicfoundation.com

Disclaimer:
The findings/views/opinions expressed in this book are solely those of the author and do not necessarily reflect the views of the publisher.

Cataloging in Publication Data--DK
Courtesy: D.K. Agencies (P) Ltd. <docinfo@dkagencies.com>

Sharma, Rekha.
Quantifying under-nutrition in rural India / Rekha Sharma.
p. cm.
Includes bibliographical references (p.).
ISBN 9789332700147

1. Malnutrition--India. 2. Ingestion--India. I. Title.

DDC 363.80954 23

Typeset by Italics India, New Delhi.

Printed and bound by The Book Mint, New Delhi.
www.thebookmint.in

Contents

List of Tables and Figures

Tables

Figures

Foreword

The discussion on malnutrition among young children in India is now part of the mainstream academic and public policy discourses. The paradox of decades of economic growth not having translated into commensurate improvements in physical indicators of well-being—including childhood stunting, underweight and anaemia—is now receiving a lot of attention, including the setting up of a separate unit within the Prime Minister's office to address this issue. This was not, however, always the case: until recently food security and nutrition security were considered synonymous. Even today, the country's food security interventions focus far more on the quantity of food, rather than its quality, and are not completely integrated with nutritional outcomes.

Dr Sharma's research, presented in this book, was amongst the earliest (if not the earliest) studies to document the extent of micronutrient malnutrition—a reflection of poor quality of diets—and the extent to which they appear responsive to income in rural India. Using the nationally-representative data on consumption expenditure for over a lakh households, she has tracked over time changes in the composition of diet, focusing not just on calories, protein and fat, but the first ever quantification of the intake of principal micronutrients in rural India. Another first to her credit is that her study was the first to point out the decreasing consumption of cereals as the primary explanation for the decline in iron intakes in India. Her research has also highlighted the seasonal nature of pattern of inadequacy, which is far lower in the months when vegetables, fruits and milk—all rich sources of micronutrients—are plentiful.

Her analysis of the determinants of dietary quality, and its relationship to manifestations of anaemia is exemplary, as is the careful way in which she has accounted for other factors that might affect these relationships, including availability of sanitation and access to health care. This is particularly welcome, given the current preference to search for magic bullets to address an inherently complex issue. Although her data set pertains primarily to the 1980s and 1990s, her analysis and its implications remain relevant even today.

This book is based on the research that Dr Sharma conducted as part of her doctoral dissertation at the Delhi School of Economics, University of Delhi. I am glad to see that Academic Foundation has seen fit to bring this research to the reach of a much wider audience.

J.V. Meenakshi
Professor, Department of Economics
Delhi School of Economics

Acknowledgements

A research work of this kind draws sustenance from several sources. Among all, an unstinted support from supervisors prominently stands out. I would like to express my deepest sense of gratitude to Prof J.V. Meenakshi and (late) Prof Sanghamitra Das for guiding this research project and taking it to its culmination. Without their continuous unflinching support, invaluable guidance, unending inspiration and generous contribution of time, it would have been well-nigh impossible for me to have accomplished this task.

My sincere thanks are due to Prof Jean Dreze for his invaluable suggestions at my pre-submission seminar. I immensely benefitted therefrom.

I would like to convey my special thanks to Prof K.L. Krishna, Prof K. Sundaram, Prof P.B. Nayak, Prof T.C. Anant, Prof Abhijit Banerjee and Prof Ashwini Deshpande for their guidance and generous help. Prof S.C. Panda, head of the academic fraternity, was ever willing to extend his moral support which I so badly needed.

I owe a word of thanks and appreciation to the staff of Centre of Development Economics and Ratan Tata Library. Mr Sanjeev Sharma and Mr K.P. Vinayan deserve my special thanks for extending their help in data handling and processing.

Dr Jaspal Singh, Principal, Sri Guru Gobind Singh College of Commerce, was a real morale-booster and came to my rescue in critical times. He has been a tremendous source of strength.

I am thankful to UGC for providing me grant under the minor research project scheme.

I am also grateful to M.S. Swaminathan Research Foundation, United Nations World Food Programme, and the Food and Agricultural Organisation for allowing me to present the preliminary results as, 'Micronutrient Deficiencies in Rural Diets' in the conference, "Towards Hunger Free India" in April 2003. Later, it became a part of the book, *Towards Hunger Free India: From Vision to Action*.

Needless to say, a researcher needs support from all corners. It is especially true of married females and I am no exception. My entire family stood rocklike behind me ungrudgingly. My two kids who had to forego many comforts in their formative periods deserve a special mention. It is the love and affection of my husband, Dr Pankaj Sharma, and my children, Vyom and Manasvi, that gave me the strength during this difficult grind.

I owe the entire thesis to my late mother-in-law who shouldered my responsibilities despite her illness. My father-in-law, Prof R.A. Sharma, has been another supervisor for me. I think without his encouragement, I would have never thought of venturing into this project. I really admire his patience for going through all the drafts without a grudge.

My friends and colleagues readily agreed to perform odd tasks, just to drive pleasure out of fruition of this arduous research endeavour. I am grateful to all of them.

— Rekha Sharma

1 Introduction

1.1 Context and Objectives of the Study

Nearly three decades after the achievement of self-sufficiency in food grains, with abundant stocks of grain, and substantial reductions in mortality and fertility rates, levels of malnutrition are still very high in India. More than half of children under the age of three years are underweight, 30 per cent of newborns are significantly underweight, more than one-third of women aged 15–49 years are chronically energy deficient and half are anaemic (NFHS, 1998-99). Almost half of the children who are estimated to have at least mild vitamin A deficiency (VAD) worldwide reside in India. VAD causes an estimated 60,000 children in India to go blind each year (OMNI Micronutrient Fact Sheet, 1996).

According to the surveys conducted by the National Nutrition Monitoring Bureau (NNMB) in 10 states (NNMB, 2002), 68 per cent of women and 71 per cent of children consume less than 50 per cent of the recommended daily allowance (RDA) for iron, while 86 per cent of women and 87 per cent of children consume less than 50 per cent of the RDA for vitamin A.

Traditional approaches to the study of nutrient deprivation in India have focussed on calorie deficiency using Food and Agriculture Organisation (FAO) of United Nations (UN), National Sample Survey (NSS) or NNMB data sets, and on the eradication of hunger—be it through enhancement of purchasing power, or through other interventions. However, malnutrition is much more than simply calorie deficiency. In recent years, there has been a dramatic change in the conceptualisation of the problem of malnutrition. The focus on food security has expanded to include issues related to nutrition security, which includes not just calories but proteins and micronutrients comprising vitamins and minerals as well.

As nutritionist Gopalan (2004) has pointed out, our objective should not be just 'freedom from hunger' but 'freedom from undernutrition'. He argues that what India needs is not a second green revolution but a food and agriculture policy with a nutrition orientation, which will result in increase in not only the conventional food grains but also of quality foods like pulses, green leafy vegetables, fruits, milk, meat, egg, fish, etc.

In part, this reorientation has occurred because there is evidence that over time the incidence of hunger has declined dramatically, although it has not been eliminated. Chronic hunger and the severe malnutrition associated with it may not be major problems any more. For example, according to the NSS (1983) consumer expenditure survey, in an answer to a question eliciting self-assessment about the adequacy of food, 18 per cent of rural and 6 per cent of urban households reported themselves to be hungry. Most of this hunger was seasonal in nature; the chronically hungry households were only 0.77 per cent in urban and 2.33 per cent in the rural sector (Minhas, 1991). By the 1999-2000 survey, these figures had dropped significantly.

Furthermore, during the 1987 drought, villages that were affected could maintain their consumption at the normal year levels because of stable food grain prices, enhanced public distribution supplies and availability of consumption credit (Acharya, 1989; Bidinger *et al.*, 1990).

Nevertheless, micronutrient malnutrition levels remain high in India. Due to limited availability of data on nutritional status, it is difficult to make comparisons over time. However, the evidence suggests that while the percentage of children under three years of age who are underweight has declined, yet half of such children remain underweight. Similarly, three-fourth of children under three have either mild or moderate or severe anaemia (NFHS, 1998-99).

Nutrition security encompasses food security and considers micronutrients as well. Unlike energy and protein, vitamins and minerals are required by the body in very small amounts, say in few milligrams or micrograms per day. Micronutrients are not present in all foods; rather some are present in very few. Therefore, eating more food by itself would not ensure adequate intake of micronutrients. In fact, unlike energy, the lack of which manifests as hunger, the lack of micronutrients often goes unperceived by the body. For this reason, micronutrient deprivation is also referred to as 'hidden hunger'.

The consequences of micronutrient deprivation for nutritional status are many. Deficiencies of even the small amounts of required vitamins and minerals can lead to serious consequences in terms of weakened immunity system, poor cognitive development, lower productivity as adults and greater susceptibility to diet related chronic diseases. Particularly vulnerable are preschool children and pregnant women but deficiencies are debilitating for all age groups. Undernourished female children are likely to become undernourished women and in turn are more likely to give birth to undernourished babies, thus perpetuating the intergenerational transmission of deprivation.

Iron deficiency anaemia can cause chronic ill health, such as impaired fetal development during pregnancy, delayed cognitive development and increased risk of infection in young children, and reduced physical capacity in all people. A shortage of riboflavin, a member of B-vitamins, may manifest itself as cracks and sores at the corners of the mouth, eye disorders, inflammation of the mouth and tongue, skin lesions, poor digestion, retarded growth, and slow mental responses. Xerophthalmia (dry eye) is the manifestation of VAD that can lead to blindness.

It has been estimated that in India, deficiencies in iron, vitamin A and iodine alone cause economic losses at least $10 billion annually in terms of lost productivity, illness, and lower physical and mental performance and death (World Bank, 1994). More recent estimates suggest that the burden of iron deficiency in India amounts to an annual loss of the equivalent of 0.4 per cent of GDP (Stein *et al.*, 2005).

In the Indian context, there are limited studies focussing on micronutrient deprivation and its determinants. Nor are the consequences of micronutrient deprivation in terms of adverse nutritional status, and their determinants, well understood.

Much of the work in India has been limited to calorie intakes and their distribution across income groups (both at aggregate and state level). For example, Meenakshi and Vishwanathan (2001) and Radhakrishna and Ravi (1992) highlight the decline in calorie intake over time. These studies also draw attention towards sharp divergence between poverty estimates based on income and calorie deprivation and point to the need to go beyond the income based poverty estimates (Palmer-Jones and Sen, 2001; Meenakshi and Vishwanathan, 2003).

Other studies attempting to quantify the extent of micronutrient deficiencies in India have typically focused on its clinical (NFHS, 1998-1999) and sub-clinical manifestations (Mason *et al.*, 2001); studies that systematically quantify the magnitude of deprivation in nutrient intakes *vis-à-vis* RDAs are rare. Exceptions include Shariff and Mallick (1999) who quantify calcium and iron intakes for 1993-94 using the NSS and surveys conducted by the NNMB, however these have limited geographical coverage.

This study attempts to contribute to this limited literature by analysing the correlates of nutrient intakes and nutritional status in rural India. The lessons learnt have important implications for policy interventions in the area of public health. With this end in view the study aims at, inter alia, the following objectives:

- Provide estimates of the quantum of intake of, as well as deprivation in, macronutrients—calorie, protein, fat and micronutrients—vitamin A, vitamin B (thiamine, niacin, and riboflavin), vitamin C, iron, in rural India and among 15 major states.[1]
- Examine how the macro and micronutrient intakes vary with income and how these are conditioned by education, occupational structure, household size and composition, seasonality, social status; and
- Examine how the nutritional status of children under the age of three years varies with the nutrient intake levels, socioeconomic variables and environmental factors. And also identify the key factors that are associated with prevalence of underweight and anaemia among women and young children.

This is perhaps the first comprehensive analysis of micronutrient malnutrition in rural India.

The two rich data sets used in this study are the all India surveys on consumer expenditure conducted by the National Sample Survey Organisation (NSSO) in 1983 and 1999-2000 and National Family Health Survey (NFHS) in 1998-99 for rural India. The NFHS collects information

1. Iodine deficiency is also a major public health problem in India. Approximately 150 million people are at the risk of iodine deficiency disorders; it is not included in this thesis because till recently, no reliable figures for iodine content of Indian food were available (Gopalan *et al.*, 2004) and it is mainly found in sea food.

with regard to nutritional status for ever-married women between 15-49 years and children under the age of 3 years only.

1.2 An Approach to the Problem

As a first step to the analysis, we quantify intakes of six micronutrients—vitamin B (thiamine, riboflavin, and niacin), vitamin A (carotene), vitamin C, iron and three macronutrients—calories, proteins and fat intakes. We compute nutrient intakes by using the information on consumption of food items from unit record data of the NSS rounds 1983 and 1999-2000 and nutrient content from food composition tables. This information is also disaggregated by state and income levels—for 15 major states and 4 quartiles. This is the first time micronutrient intakes have been quantified for India using a nationally representative data set.

We then calculate incidence, depth and severity of nutrient deprivation in terms of Foster-Greer-Thorbecke (FGT) class of indices, between 1983 and 1999-2000. In computing these, instead of following the traditional practice of using the same RDA for all individuals, we use information with respect to the age and sex composition of the household to compute the RDAs of different nutrients at the household level. These FGT indices do not explain any causal relationship but are a useful descriptive tool, and provide the context for understanding the correlates of nutrient intakes and nutritional status.

That there is a need to go beyond considering the determinants of nutrient intakes to consider indicators of nutritional status is underscored by the apparent weak correlation, at least at the state level, between nutrient intakes and health outcomes. For example, if we look at nutritional status as measured in terms of anthropometric measures or anaemia, we find that the southern states of Kerala, Tamil Nadu and Andhra Pradesh have lower calorie intakes but these states rank high and perform better in terms of health outcomes as compared to Punjab and Haryana. The relationship between income and nutritional status is also not strong. States with high prevalence rates of anaemia among children and among women include richer states such as Punjab, Haryana, as well as the poor states of Bihar and Orissa (NFHS, 1998-99). Also crucial in determining nutritional status is the absorption of nutrient intakes or bioavailability of the nutrient (rather than nutrient ingested), which significantly depends on the living environment.

Figure 1.1 presents a schematic representation of a conceptual framework within which these objectives may be addressed. The framework, adapted and modified from that outlined in Smith and Haddad (2000), distinguishes nutritional status from nutrient intakes. Both are influenced by income, demographic factors, education and factors associated with the living environment. Further, nutrient intakes also influence nutritional status.

Figure 1.1

Conceptual Framework Used in Empirical Analysis for Determination of Nutritional Status

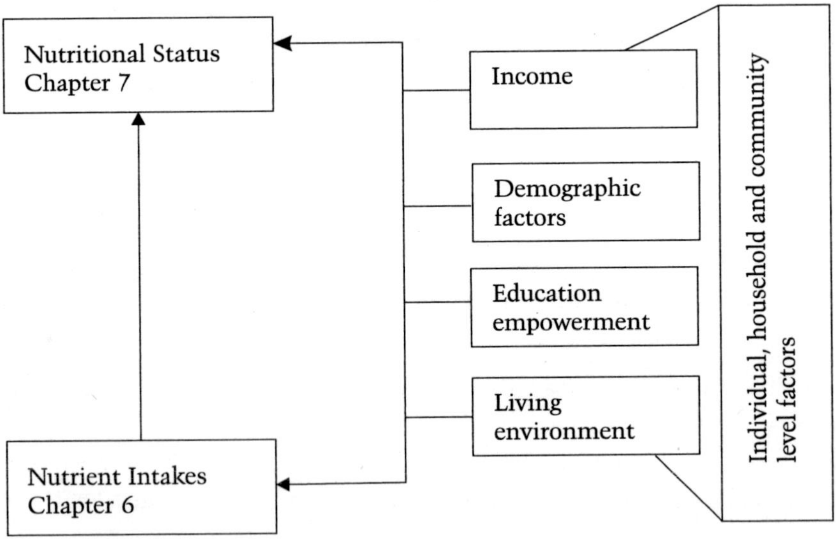

Consider first, the lower left box in Figure 1.1, nutrient intakes and their correlates. The motivation for analysing the effect of income on nutrient intake is provided by the lack of consensus among researchers on the magnitude of income elasticity of nutrient intakes. Some economists have found these nutrient–expenditure elasticities to be insignificant as increases in income may translate into an increase in price per calorie consumed without a corresponding increase in nutrient intake, a reflection of the preference for variety over quantity. Even the Indian evidence is mixed. Behrman and Deolalikar (1987), using International Crops Research Institute for the Semi-arid Tropics (ICRISAT) data for villages of rural south India, found that the income elasticity of demand for calories is statistically not different from zero. However, Subramanian and Deaton (1996), Meenakshi and Vishwanathan (2001) and Subramanian (2001) using NSS data suggest otherwise.

As indicated in Figure 1.1, demographic characteristics such as the size and composition of the household also have a significant impact on the availability of nutrients: for example, there may be economies of scale in consumption. Similarly, the nature of employment has an important bearing on nutrient intake independent of its effect through income. However, the role of occupational status in determining micronutrient intakes has not been extensively explored in literature.

Education is believed to play a major role in influencing nutritional intake. It improves the understanding of the concept of nutrition and nutritive value of food. The role of education has been well documented in literature though few studies consider the effect of education on nutrients other than energy. In case of rural India, Roy (2001) found that the coefficient of education was insignificant as rural Indian dietary habits were largely dictated by tradition than by nutritional information. The pattern of consumption within the household is also influenced by who has decision-making power in the family.

Similarly, the living environment can also affect nutrient intakes, not just in determining requirements but also by their impact on the exposure to infectious diseases.

Thus, for the second objective of this thesis, using rural NSS data of 1983 and 1999-2000, we estimate a set of nine nutrient demand functions as functions of income, occupational status of household, sub-rounds, household size and composition, education, social status and head of the household. Data limitations preclude consideration of all the variables considered above.

The third objective is to explore the determinants of nutritional status. Adequate nutrient intakes are a necessary but not a sufficient condition for positive nutritional status.[2] Dietary intake must be adequate in quantity and quality so that the body absorbs nutrients consumed. As before, the income variable captures the potential to achieve resources for food and other basic needs. In addition, the availability of caregivers and their quality also influence the nutritional status of children. These factors include the number of children who compete for household resources, the mother's autonomy in decision-making, and her knowledge and beliefs. In addition to resources for care, the living environment, which comprises availability of safe water, sanitation, shelter and health care, affect nutritional status. More details of these interactions are provided in Chapters 2 and 4.

Using the basic framework of Behrman and Skoufias (2004), Strauss and Thomas (1995), Alderman (1990), Sahn (1990), Behrman and Wolfe (1982; 1987a), Pitt and Rosenzweig (1985) etc., we have assumed that nutritional status is the output of the production function that has its inputs as nutrient intakes and the four categories of non-nutrient factors as depicted in Figure 1.1. Nutritional status can thus be viewed as the outcome of a provisioning process with inputs of food, non-food commodities, services and care.

These factors may also be categorised as individual, parent, household and community level variables following Mosley and Chen (1984), Schultz (1984) and others. Nutrient intakes, and demographic characteristics such as age, gender and birth order of the child, age of the mother, are individual-level factors. Parental education and autonomy in the household decision-making also affect the ability to provide care and are parent-level factors. The living environment is important both at the household and community levels and is represented by the type of house, source of water, provision of sanitation facilities at the household level, and accessibility to health facilities and sewerage system at the community level.

Thus, in the first part of this objective, using a fixed effect specification, we analyse the impact of these variables on standardised weight-for-age, an indicator of the nutritional status of the children under three years of age.

---

2. Some studies postulate a simultaneous determination of nutrient intakes and nutritional outcomes; instead, the framework above highlights the pathways through which nutritional status is influenced.

Since the NFHS data used for this exercise do not contain information on micronutrient intakes, therefore, in the second part of the exercise, exploiting the near-coincidence of the NSS survey in 1999-2000 and the NFHS survey in 1998-99, we merge the two data sets for rural India with the NSS region as the unit of observation. Using this data set, we employ canonical correlation techniques to identify the key factors that are associated with prevalence of underweight and anaemia among women, and children under three years of age.

1.3 Organisation of the Study

Chapter 1 presents an overview of the problem of malnutrition. Chapter 2 presents a review of literature on nutrient demand functions and its determinants. It also reviews the role of dietary intakes and other social, economic and environmental variables in determining nutritional status. Chapter 3 describes the two data sets, namely all India consumer expenditure surveys (NSS) and NFHS used in the study. It also discusses the third set which has been created by merging these two data sets at the regional level for rural India. It gives a brief account of the food composition tables and recommended dietary allowance figures used in this study.

Chapter 4 presents the methodology used to assess trends in micronutrient deprivation, and the techniques used to estimate determinants of nutrient demand and the correlates of nutritional status.

A discussion on trends in food consumption and dietary diversification finds a place in Chapter 5 and quantifies nutrient deprivation in rural India and among 15 major states across quartiles. The role of income and other correlates of nutrient intakes are discussed in Chapter 6. Chapter 7 studies the relationship between nutrient intakes, other socioeconomic variables and nutritional status. Finally, the principal results and their policy implications are presented in Chapter 8.

2 Review of Literature

This chapter reviews available studies on issues regarding nutrition and nutritional status, and the determinants of nutrient intakes (section 2.2) and nutritional status (section 2.3). To provide a context for the evidence presented later, section 2.1 briefly discusses the studies on dietary changes in India.

2.1 Changes in the Diet Composition

With economic development, changes in food habits are expected. By Engel's law, food shares decline; also, by Bennet's law, consumers typically switch to a more expensive diet, substituting quality for quantity (Bennett, 1954). In particular, the starchy staple ratio and the percentage of calories derived from cereals and cereal substitute declines with economic growth, and the consumption of vegetables, fruits, milk and meat increases. This transformation of the diet has occurred in India as well. Although varied in nature and focus, various studies *viz.*, Subramanian (2001), Chelliah and Sudershan (1999), Shariff and Mallick (1999), Meenakshi (1996), Subramanian and Deaton (1996), Suryanarayana (1995) and Radhakrishna and Ravi (1992), testify to this change for India.

According to nutritionists, dietary diversity is a key element of this transformation to high-quality diets (Ruel, 2003). Therefore, it is expected that with changes in the dietary pattern, nutrient intakes should improve. In this research work, to see if any dietary diversification has been witnessed in rural Indian diets between 1983 and 1999-2000, we calculate the dietary diversity index and also compute percentage of households consuming different commodities.

2.2 Studies on Nutrient Demand Functions

Studies that have analysed the determinants of nutrient intakes have either followed the approach: (i) of estimating food demand/expenditure systems and then converting the price and income elasticities into nutrient elasticities using fixed food-nutrient conversion factors (Strauss, 1984; Pitt, 1983; Murty and Radhakrishna, 1981) or (ii) estimating directly the demand for nutrients as function of food prices, household size, per capita expenditure, etc. (Lancaster *et al.*, 2004; Gibson and Rozelle, 2002; Meenakshi and Vishwanathan, 2001; Roy, 2001; Subramanian and Deaton, 1996; Behrman and Deolalikar, 1987; Behrman and Wolfe, 1984).

2.2.1 Income

The literature has seen intensive discussion on the role of income in increasing the intake of nutrients, especially calories as it has important policy implications.

One widely held view is that malnutrition will disappear only with the improvements in income that accompany the development process. The World Bank (1980: 59) articulates this view forcefully, "Malnutrition is largely a reflection of poverty; people do not have income for food. Given the slow increase in income that is likely for the poorest people in the foreseeable future, large numbers will remain malnourished for decades to come. The most efficient long-term policies are those that raise the income of the poor..."

This view is supported by many studies that report a high elasticity (and sometimes close to unity) of nutrient intake, especially calories with respect to income—0.82 for rural Sierra Leone (Strauss, 1982), 0.8 for rural Bangladesh (Pitt, 1983), 0.51 for rural Indonesia (Timmer and Alderman, 1979), 0.24-0.5 for Northern Brazil (Ward and Sanders, 1980), to name a few examples.

However Behrman and Deolalikar (1987), challenged this view. Using International Crops Research Institute for the Semi-arid Tropics (ICRISAT) data for villages of south India, their pioneer study estimated that income elasticity of demand for calories was very low and statistically not very different from zero. Thus, they concluded, household income may not have much effect on total calorie intake and additional expenditure was incurred on the other non-nutritive attributes of food.

Others like Bouis and Novenario-Reese (1997), Bouis and Haddad (1992), Bhargava (1991a), Bouis (1990), Ravallion (1990), Strauss and Thomas (1990) and Behrman and Wolfe (1984) also suggested that these elasticities are typically less than 0.20 and often insignificant. Some of these studies and some of the estimated elasticity are mentioned in Table 2.1.

Table 2.1

Some Calorie Expenditure Elasticity Estimates

Author	*Country*	*Year*	*Elasticity (at mean)*
Ward and Sanders	Brazil	1980	0.24-0.53
Pitt	Bangladesh	1983	0.78-82
Behrman and Wolfe	Nicaragua	1984	0.05
Strauss	Sierra Leone	1984	0.82
Alderman	India	1987	0.41-0.44
Behrman and Deolalikar	India	1987	0.17-0.37
Timmer and Alderman	Indonesia (rural)	1987	0.51
Timmer and Alderman	Indonesia (urban)	1987	0.26
Sahn	Sri Lanka	1988	0.62
Von Braun	Guatemala	1989	0.31
Ravallion	Indonesia	1990	0.15
Strauss and Thomas	Brazil	1990	0.11-0.20
Bhargava	India	1991	0.05
Bouis and Haddad	Philippines	1992	0.08-0.14
Subramanian and Deaton	India	1994	0.37
Bouis and Novenario-Reese	Bangladesh	1997	0.18
Skoufias	Indonesia	2001	0.32-0.45
Roy	India	2001	0.10
Gibson and Rozelle	Papua New Guinea (urban)	2002	0.60

The issue of variability of the calorie-expenditure elasticity across income groups has been widely discussed in the literature as marginal responses to income changes are likely to be much higher for the lower income groups than for the rich (Ravallion, 1990; Strauss and Thomas, 1995). Therefore, elasticities reported at mean incomes may not be relevant for the poor and undernourished group. Further, as incomes increase, there is substitution between the food groups that lead to a fall in the elasticity. Strauss and Thomas (1990) have estimated the calorie expenditure elasticity for urban Brazil for the upper and the lower quartile to be 0.02 and 0.26 respectively.

The issue of non-linearities in the income response has also been explored for India and its states. Meenakshi and Ray (1999) have suggested that inclusion of a quadratic income term is appropriate in the Indian case. Meenakshi and Vishwanathan (2001) have estimated the calorie and protein elasticities for different quartiles of Indian population. They have a significant negative quadratic parameter of income in the nutrient demand function, implying fall in the elasticity with income.

The issue of non-linearities has also been examined using non-parametric techniques (Gibson and Rozelle, 2002; Skoufias, 2001; Roy 1996, 2001; Subramanian, 2001; Subramanian and Deaton, 1996). These studies indicate that income elasticities do change with income level and are high at low levels of income.

Other Nutrient Elasticities

Though much of the empirical work has been restricted to calorie-expenditure elasticity, some studies have also considered protein, fat and micronutrients. These studies indicate that income elasticities are of magnitude of 0.6 to 0.8 for proteins in rural Bangladesh (Pitt, 1983) and 0.3 to 0.5 for North Eastern Brazil (Ward and Sanders, 1980). However, Behrman and Wolfe (1984) suggest that for Nicaragua income elasticities for protein, iron and vitamin A are small in magnitude, i.e., 0.04, 0.10, and 0.07 respectively.

Bouis and Novenario-Reese (1997) need a special mention as they measure the magnitude of income responses for five major nutrients *viz.*, calories, fat, iron, vitamin A and vitamin C for 1991-92 in Bangladesh. They find that the coefficient of income is significantly greater than zero for calorie, fat, vitamin C and iron, only exception being vitamin A. The elasticity for calories, iron, vitamin C and fat is estimated to be 0.18, 0.27, 0.81 and 1.21 respectively. The fat elasticity is high because of high-income elasticity of cooking oil and other food products associated with it. In general, it supports the fact that elasticity of the nutrient depends on the elasticity of the good from which it is mainly derived.

Similarly, Meenakshi and Vishwanathan (2001) have estimated calorie and protein elasticity for rural Indian states for 1983 and 1993-94 and find that just like calorie elasticities, protein elasticities are non-zero, range between 0.4 to 0.5 on an average and decline with income. Further, these elasticities have declined over time in most of the states.

Lancaster *et al.* (2004) have estimated expenditure elasticities for calorie, protein and fat for rural areas in few Indian states and found them to be significantly different from zero.

Various reasons have been put forward to explain for the difference in the magnitude of nutrient expenditure elasticities. Firstly, elasticity estimates are affected by the fact whether these are obtained directly from calorie demand functions or indirect conversions from food demand equations. As Bouis (1994) and Behrman and Deolalikar (1987) point out, high calorie elasticities are the result of applying constant conversion factors to broad food groups to obtain calorie or nutrient consumed. It does not take into account quality of food consumed. These indirect nutrient elasticities with respect to expenditure overstate the true elasticities as there are possibilities of intra-group substitution. For example, Pitt (1983) and Murthy and Radhakrishna (1981) used only nine food groups and Strauss (1982) used only five groups. An indirect calorie expenditure elasticity of 0.77 was four and a half times higher than directly estimated calorie elasticity of 0.17, as calculated by Behrman and Deolalikar (1987), for India.

Secondly, the fact that household expenditures (used as a proxy for income), an independent variable and nutrient intake, the dependent variable, are determined from the same household consumption data set introduces a bias in the estimation of nutrient expenditure elasticity. The error in the nutrient intake equation would be correlated with household expenditure and thus, may bias the elasticity estimates upwards as discussed by Bouis and Haddad (1992). While the resulting bias may be reduced through the use of instruments, in general, it is very difficult to find a set of instruments which are correlated with income but not with errors in the measurement.

Thirdly, measurement error bias is likely to be introduced if household resources are measured by income rather than expenditure because there are more fluctuations in current income than expenditure (Bhalotra and Atfield, 1998).

Thus, for India, while there are studies quantifying income elasticities of demand for macronutrients, there has been no such attempt for micronutrients. This study may perhaps be a pacesetter in this regard.

2.2.2 Occupational Structure

The nature of employment has an important bearing on nutrient intake, independent of its effect through income. Therefore, the type of economic activity being undertaken may influence food consumption, thus nutrient intake. Further, the physical requirement of energy depends on the kind of activity undertaken by workers. It is usually postulated that rural workers on an average require more energy than urban workers since they do more physical work. Pitt (1983) found significant differences in the behaviour of cultivator and non-cultivator houscholds in Bangladcsh.

Using National Sample Survey (NSS) data for rural Maharashtra for 1983, Subramanian and Deaton (1996) have found that average calorie intake of self-employed non-agricultural households and non-agricultural labour households does not differ from that of other labour households. However, self-employed agricultural households and agricultural labour households have higher calorie intake than other labour households.

The role of occupational status in determining nutrient demand, especially of micronutrients, has not been extensively studied in the literature. In this study, we introduce occupational structure dummy variables (as per NSS classification) as explanatory variables to examine their impact on nutrient intakes.

2.2.3 Seasonality

Agricultural work by its very nature is seasonal. This seasonality in earnings may, in turn, be reflected in seasonality of nutrient intake, the contrast between peak and lean seasons being of particular interest. Bouis and Haddad (1992) and Ravallion (1990) suggest that there are seasonal fluctuations in calorie intake. Behrman (1988a) also suggests that factors governing allocation of nutrients among children differ significantly across seasons.

Using Indian NSS data for 1983 and 1991-92, Meenakshi and Vishwanathan (2001) analysed the seasonal fluctuations in calories and protein intake through seasonal dummies in the nutrient Engel demand functions. They concluded that there is no significant seasonality in the calories and protein intake as a result of seasonality in production. They suggest that extent of seasonality has declined overtime.

A priori, it would be expected that consumers would possibly protect calorie intake from seasonality through consumption smoothing of staple foods. This is not necessarily possible with nutrients like vitamin A, vitamin C, whose main sources do not lie in staple foods like wheat, rice, but in few foods such as vegetables and fruits whose production is much more seasonal in nature and that do not store as easily as the staples.

Bouis and Novenario-Reese (1997) have reported much more seasonality in the intake of vitamin A, vitamin C and iron whose source is concentrated in few seasonal vegetables and fruits than calories and fat in Bangladesh in 1991-92.

This study examines whether the same can be said of micronutrients in India.

2.2.4 Household Size and Composition

Both size and composition of a household influence per capita food expenditure. Deaton and Paxson (1998) find that at constant per capita total expenditure, the per capita demand for food decreases with household size. The explanation is economies of scale—arising on account of bulk purchases, bulk preparation of food, less wastage through better management, lowering of overhead costs, etc. Therefore, we might expect the presence of economies of scale to imply that larger households with same level of income are better off than smaller households.

Behrman and Wolfe (1984) found a significantly negative coefficient for household size in the nutrient demand functions for calorie, protein, iron and vitamin A.

Subramanian and Deaton (1996) estimated separate calorie Engel curves for households of different sizes. They conclude that the elasticity of calories with respect to expenditure is not much affected by the size of household, as different regression lines are approximately parallel to each other. But the curves are lower for larger households, so that conditional on total expenditure, calorie consumption per capita falls with household size—an effect that is at least partly due to the fact that larger households have larger proportion of children.

While a relationship between calories per head and total expenditure per head is a natural starting point and allows for household size in a rough way, it makes no allowance for the fact that children consume fewer calories than their parents.

Adult equivalent units are often used to account for household composition. For example, a male in the age group 20-39 years is considered the standard known as the 'reference man' and his *per diem* energy forms a single unit. The corresponding unit for adult women is 0.71. The adult equivalent units can also be calculated econometrically as in Meenakshi and Ray (1999).

Subramanian and Deaton (1996) decomposed the population into 10 age-sex group dummies, 5 each for male and female group, to study the differences in the nutritional intake among them. They also found that adults consume more than children in rural Maharashtra[1] but that there is no evidence of gender bias among children.

In this study, size and composition of households have been introduced in the traditional way to study the pattern of nutrient intake, especially micronutrients, without addressing the issue of gender biasedness in the family.

2.2.5 Social Status of Household

The status of the household largely reflects social status of the household, which has implications in terms of economic well-being. As is well documented, in India, the SC/ST community is poorer than others. Subramanian and Deaton (1996) suggest that this extends to calorie intake as well, and introduce it as one of the variables in explaining the consumption of calories. Meenakshi and Vishwanathan (2001) also introduce SC/ST variable in the nutrient demand functions and find that after controlling for income and other demographical characteristics, in

1. In case of household expenditure surveys, household composition, represented by proportion of household members belonging to the various age-sex groups, can be used to test for the possible gender bias in nutrient intakes.

most of the states, nutrient intake among the SC/ST are no different from those of other communities. In fact, in some of the states, the average calorie intake turned to be higher for SC/ST than others.

In this dissertation, we examine whether there are differences in the micronutrient intakes of the SC/ST households as compared to households belonging to other communities.

2.2.6 Education

Education is expected to enable informed choices with respect to purchases of food items as well as nutrient intakes. It is believed to play a major role in influencing nutritional intake as it improves the understanding of the concept of nutrition and nutritive contents of food. The empirical evidence is mixed. Ravallion (1990) finds that the calorie demand is negatively related to the level of schooling of the head of the family in Indonesia. He suggests that the possible reason for this perverse sign may be lower energy requirements for jobs performed by highly educated people. Using household data from Nicaragua, Behrman and Wolfe (1984) find that educated women may be better informed about the nutritional content of food, importance of good nutrition and the product options available. Therefore, they can hold a stronger decision-making position in the household. The study indicates that schooling of women has positive effects on all nutrient intakes.

Pitt and Rosenzwig (1985) and Ward and Sanders (1980), however, find no significant effect of woman's schooling on household nutrient consumption.

Roy (2001) introduces education level of the wife of the household head as a variable affecting nutritional status of the Indian household. It is found that education is not significant. She suggests that this may be because of very low level of literacy and the fact that rural Indian dietary habits are normally dictated by tradition rather than by nutritional information.

Very few studies consider the effect of education on nutrients other than energy. Bouis and Novenario-Reese (1997) report perverse negative sign, but insignificant for level of education of the househead in the nutrient demand functions of calories, iron, vitamin A and vitamin C for Bangladesh. However, fat demand function has statistically significant negative value. Behrman and Wolfe (1984) indicate that the households in which women have more schooling tend to be significantly better nourished, *ceteris paribus*, particularly in regard to consuming yellow and green leafy vegetables and other foods rich in vitamin A.

In our study, we introduce a dummy variable representing households with at least one adult literate member to test its importance in explaining macro and micronutrient intakes.

2.2.7 Head of the Household

Nutrient intakes may also be influenced by whether the head of the family is female or male. Assuming that women are better informed about preparation and contents of food, female-headed households are likely to have higher micronutrient intakes than in households where women do not influence the purchase and decisions of the household.

Bouis and Novenario-Reese (1997) found that there is no significant difference in the vitamin A, vitamin C and fat intake between male or female-headed households in Bangladesh.

This study would make a contribution by studying the effect of head of the household on macro as well as micronutrient intakes.

2.2.8 Issues Related to Measurement and Concept

The method of data collection also affects the magnitude of nutrient intakes and elasticities. One method used is to estimate nutrient availability from household consumption surveys. The other method is to conduct nutrition surveys, that is, obtain information on nutrient intakes rather than nutrient availability by collecting data on actual food consumed over the reference period. It is argued that it is more precise to actually measure the amount of food consumed rather than ask the respondent to aggregate over the reference period.

The length of recall period with regard to food intake also influences the magnitude of nutrients. Though the 24 hourly recall data commonly used in nutrition monitoring surveys may give precise information, these are probably noisier because of day-to-day variation in food consumed. Further, these are very intensive and expensive ways to collect data on consumption.

Therefore, household consumption surveys based on food purchases remain more popular.

In calculating nutrient intake, meals eaten outside the home as well as meals served to guests must be taken into account. For example, calorie availability may exceed calorie intake for the richer households who give out meals to servants and employees and reverse for the poor who receive meals or free gifts from others. Therefore, uncorrected wastages and leakages would bias the nutrient estimates as indicated in the work of Subramanian and Deaton (1996), Bouis and Haddad (1992) and Minhas (1991). Therefore, a distinction needs to be made between nutrient availability and nutrient intake for an individual. In this dissertation, meals are not accounted for, as it is difficult to estimate the micronutrient content of such meals.

In addition to issues relating to the measurement of nutrient intake, the use of nutrient norms has also been addressed in the literature. The derived nutrient intake for each household is usually compared with a nutritional norm. Nutrient requirements vary between households according to their size, sex, age and work activity. Further, it has been argued that the human regulatory mechanism allows energy expenditure to adapt to changes in nutritional intake such that the very existence of fixed requirement level for any reference household is unlikely. Rather, there exist multiple intake equilibria at which body weight is locally maintained, although there are biological limits to adaptation. The possibilities of sustained downward adaptation clearly become negligible at low intake expenditure equilibria. These issues have been discussed in detail in section 4.1.

Within the limitations of data as mentioned above, we use the monthly food expenditure data to get estimates of per household per day nutrient availability. These household estimates have been compared to recommended daily allowance for the household which accounts for demographic composition of the household.

2.3 Studies on Nutritional Status Production Function

There is a limited but growing literature, which focusses attention not just on nutrient intakes—an input indicator, but also on nutritional status of the population—output indicator, especially women and children—the most vulnerable groups. In this section, we review a number of issues regarding the measurement of nutritional status and studies focussing on the correlates of nutritional status.

Nutritional status is generally captured by anthropometric measures of height, weight, triceps, skinfold thickness, or nutritional deficiencies based on biochemical (serum/plasma) tests. These measures differ significantly in regard to their cost and measurement error. Anthropometric measurements are easy and less expensive than biochemical measures.

Weight and height are the most commonly used (Payne, 1992; Waterlow, 1984) as compared to triceps, skinfold thickness, etc., and nutritional deficiencies like anaemia, vitamin A deficiency, etc., as compared to per capita intake of food. Data on height and weight are used to calculate the three summary indices: weight-for-age, height-for-age and weight-for-height. These indices are also expressed in standard deviation units (z-score) from the median for the international reference population. Children who are more than two standard deviations below the reference median on any of the indices are considered to be undernourished, and children who fall more than three standard deviations below the reference median are considered to be severely undernourished. The three common anthropometric indicators available are as follows:

(a) Weight-for-age: When a child does not receive sufficient and adequate food relative to his needs, is ill, or both, his body weight may be temporarily reduced. If the situation causing low weight is rectified, the child will catch up. A low weight-for-age is also called underweight.

(b) Height-for-age: If the episodes of nutritional deprivation and/or disease are repeated and/or prolonged, the result may be growth failure (short height, or stunting). Stunting is a biological adaptation to inadequate food and/or frequent infection during the first few years of life and usually means that survivors face irreversible slower growth and smaller adult body size (Payne and Lipton, 1994). Stunting reflects the cumulative impact of inadequate nutrition, prolonged illness, or both—children that are often sick do not eat much and do not grow tall. It is still not entirely resolved that what role genetic factors play for human height and growth. But most of the studies have found that the average height of a population is largely determined by nutrition and health.

(c) Weight-for-height: Low weight relative to height is often referred to as temporary malnutrition or wasting. It reflects a recent and substantial weight loss, usually as a consequence of acute starvation and/or severe disease.

Out of the three indices available in the literature, we have chosen weight-for-age as anthropometric indicator of children under the age of three years. It is the most common indicator of anthropometric failure used in the literature. Those with low weight-for-age represent both acute as well as chronically malnourished or deprived in health care. Secondly, the problems associated with the measurement of height are much more than weight as it requires proper position/posture of the body which may be more difficult for children under three years of age. Further, for rural India, almost half of the children under three years of age are underweight and stunted (NFHS, 1998-99).

The use of anthropometric measurement to assess the nutritional status of adults as compared to children under the age of five years is rather a recent phenomenon. The two main anthropometric indicators available for adults are height and weight. Using the two measures, a body mass index (BMI) defined as weight in kilograms divided by height in meters squared (kg/m^2) is constructed. Micozzi *et al.* (1986) have shown that BMI is a better indicator of anthropometric failure than height or weight individually. Therefore, we choose BMI as an indicator of nutritional status of adults instead of any other measure. The most recent estimate of acceptable BMI is 18.5 (FAO, 1996). Therefore, an adult with BMI equal to 18.5 is consistent with health and functional fitness (Svedberg, 2002).

While there is a large biomedical literature which explores the determinants of nutritional status of the population using experimental designs, our focus here is primarily but not exclusively on the socio-economic literature. As noted in Chapter 1, the basic framework assumes nutritional status (anthropometric outcome) as the output of the production function which has as its inputs—nutrient intake and non-nutrient health related consumption goods.

Further, these determinants can be also classified into individual (child), parent, household and village specific factors.

2.3.1 Individual-Specific Factors

Nutrient Intake

The importance of adequacy of food in the determination of nutritional status of children as well as adults is well understood. Gibson and Rozelle (2002), Wolfe and Behrman (1982; 1987), Martorell and Ho (1984) and Clark (1981) use primarily energy intake (or protein) as a measure of dietary intake in case of adults, while some studies such as that of Pitt and Rosezweig (1985) have considered the role of micronutrient intakes (indicative of dietary quality) in determining the nutritional status. Controlled experimental studies of Ramakrishnan *et al.* (2004), Demment *et al.* (2003) and Rivera *et al.* (2003) emphasise the need to consider multiple micronutrients—vitamin A and C, iron and zinc—simultaneously than individually—especially in improving anthropometric outcomes.

The diet requirements, source and frequency differ for children at different ages—while exclusive breast milk is generally recommended for children upto 6 months, introduction of weaning foods is recommended from 4-6 months onwards. Inadequate and inappropriate food leads to malnourishment in the form of stunted growth, ill development of mental faculties, etc.; and it has been evident in works of Onyango *et al.* (1998), Melville *et al.* (1988) and Martorell *et al.* (1984).

Magnani *et al.* (1985), Ferguson *et al.* (1981), Clark (1981), Chandra (1979), Taylor *et al.* (1978) and Chernichovsky and Kielmann (1977) estimate health production functions for infants and young children and find significant positive association between nutrient intakes/breastfeeding and nutritional status. As far as duration of breastfeeding is concerned, there is a mixed response. Longer duration of breastfeeding is positively associated with higher weight-for-age in Greiner and Latham (1981) and Melville *et al.* (1988), while a negative association is reported between these variables in Martorell *et al.* (1984) and Wolfe and Behrman (1982).

Studies find that children in developing countries grow adequately in the first part of infancy. It is the inadequate quantity and poor quality of complementary food which is the significant factor that explains subsequent faltering in growth. Girma and Genebo (2002), Yimer (2000), Underwood and Hofvander (1982) and Scrimshaw and Underwood (1980) show the importance of complementary foods in improving the anthropometric status of the children. Martorell and Habicht (1986) clearly point out that young children have quantitative and qualitative nutritional requirements that are different from those of older children and adults. Some traditional complementary foods used in developing countries provide grossly inadequate amounts of proteins and calories in relation to requirements.

The lack of a strong association between nutrient intakes and nutritional status is noted by Haddad *et al.* (1996); Alderman (1990). This may not be surprising, especially in case of adults, since nutritional status is a cumulative outcome of nutrients ingested over a long period of time while nutrient intakes are collected over short time. Even for children where lag between nutrient intakes and nutritional status is likely to be short, the relationship between the two may not always be robust because of unobserved characteristics (Maxwell *et al.*, 2000; Behrman and Wolfe, 1987).

The role of increased iron intakes and vitamin C in combating nutritional anaemia is well discussed in medical literature as well as documented empirically in the work of Bhargava *et al.* (2001) and Tseng *et al.* (1997) for Bangladesh and Russia respectively. They have devised an algorithm to calculate bioavailable iron from mixed diet (for details, see section 3.5.4). Their results show the quality of diet to be an important factor in determining bioavailable iron. The importance of vitamin A in reducing anaemia has been highlighted by Mwanri *et al.* (2000) and Schultink and Gross (1996).

As the National Family Health Survey (NFHS) data do not contain data on nutrient intakes, in studying the nutritional status of children, we have used proxies for nutrient intakes as the current breastfeeding status and frequency of complementary diet received in the form of solid mushy food, green leafy vegetables and fruits by the child in a household. To analyse the prevalence of anaemia and underweight among women and children at the regional level, the measures of nutrient intakes used are per capita intakes of calories, iron and vitamins A and C.

Age of the Child

Children's nutritional status is more sensitive to factors such as feeding/weaning practices, care and exposure to infection, especially when exclusive breastfeeding stops around 4-6 months of age. Studies by Maxwell *et al.* (2000), Yimer (2000), Samson and Lakech (2000), Genebo *et al.* (1999) and Mishra *et al.* (1999) find evidence that nutritional status has an inverted U-shaped relationship with age, with an inflection point around 12-24 months.

The age and square of child's age is introduced in this work to examine its effect on nutritional status of children.

Birth Order of the Child

Birth order of the child is another variable explaining the risk of malnourishment in children. Most of the literature suggests that younger siblings are nutritionally disadvantaged (Mishra *et al.*, 1999; Horton, 1988; Wolfe and Behrman, 1987; Bairagi, 1986). This is often explained in terms of less maternal care, cultural reasons and socioeconomic reasons (parents are more dependent on first child for their security in old age). However, studies of Melville *et al.* (1988) and Ryan *et al.* (1984) have found no significant relationship between birth order and nutritional status of children. We also examine the effect of birth order on nutritional status of the children.

Gender of the Child

Studies by Behrman (1987; 1988b) have found that male children are favoured in terms of allocation of food, health and other nutritional inputs and thus have better nutritional status, while empirical findings of Haddad (1987) and Horton (1986) indicate the bias in favour of female children. In studies of Olaniyan (2002), Maxwell *et al.* (2000), Mishra *et al.* (1999) and Melville *et al.* (1988), the sex of the child is not significantly related to nutritional status, indicating no bias towards male or female children.

In this study, we introduce a gender dummy variable and its interaction with birth order to understand its effect on nutritional status of children.

Health of the Child

Illnesses have an impact on the effective absorption and utilisation of nutrients. Frequent infections or chronic diseases affect the efficiency of nutrient utilisation of growth at the cellular level (Marotrell and Habicht,

1986). They also result in loss of appetite (Waterlow and Tomkins, 1992), and therefore, lower food intake (Martorell *et al.*, 1980) and greater waste (through excretion). Thus, there is an increased demand for nutrients to fight off infections (Svedberg, 2000).

In this research work, we have used the information on whether the child suffers from fever or diarrhoea in the past week to indicate health status of the child.

2.3.2 Parent-Specific Factors

Caregiver Resources

Care in this context is the provision (household and community) of time, attention and support to meet the physical, mental and social needs of the growing child and other household members (ICS, 1993). Studies have used different indicators of care to show their importance in determining the nutritional status. Even when there is poverty, food insecurity and limited access to health care, enhanced care within the household can produce better nutritional status.

Maxwell *et al.* (2000) have identified six major categories of human resources for care: (1) caregiver education, knowledge and beliefs; (2) caregiver health and nutritional status; (3) mental health, lack of stress and self confidence of the caregiver; (4) caregiver's autonomy and control of resources; (5) the workload and available time of caregiver; and (6) availability of alternate caregivers and social support from family and community. These human resources interact with household's economic resources, organisational resources at the community level and ideologies of the household to determine the care.

Mosley and Chen (1984) point out that the mother's skills, time and health, all operate directly on the growth and development of the child. Because of biological links between the mother and child during pregnancy and lactation, the mother's health and nutritional status influence the health and survival of the child.

In this study, we have used occupational status of the mother and father separately as variables representing caregiver resources in terms of time and resources. To represent the working status, we introduce dummy variables for different occupations *viz.*, highly skilled jobs, sales activities, agricultural labourer, self-employed in agriculture, manual skilled activities, manual unskilled activities as labourers and non-working.

Parental Education (Knowledge and Beliefs)

Parental education beyond the expected impact on productivity is associated with more efficient management of limited household resources, greater utilisation of available health care services, better health promoting behaviours, lower fertility and more child-centered caring practices—all factors associated with better child health and nutrition as evident in studies of Horton (1988), Behrman and Deolalikar (1988) and McGuire and Popkin (1989).

Education of the mother can influence the nutritional status of the child through increasing women's care giving resources and improving childcare practices involving feeding habits and personal hygiene behaviour. Maxwell *et al.* (2000) have also shown child's health begins to improve only with certain level of education of mother. Using NFHS (1992-93), Mishra *et al.* (1999) have also found mother's education to be the strongest predictor of nutritional status of children in India.

Studies by Strauss and Thomas (1995), Berhman and Wolfe (1984), Genebo *et al.* (1999) and Yimer (2000) have shown maternal education is an important determinant of nutritional status after controlling for household resources. However, other studies by Guilkey and Stewart (1995), Cebu study team (1991) or Wolfe and Behrman (1987) find a strong negative impact of maternal education on breastfeeding, especially exclusive breastfeeding because of higher value of time.

However, in the literature, another line of thought exists which argues that little variation in education levels or attending few years of school in the distant past may not make much difference to current functional abilities and thus may not help in improving the health status of the children significantly. Bhargava *et al.* (2003) modelled the role of mother's functional ability through cognitive scores rather than educational attainment and found a positive relationship cognitive scores and improved nutritional status of children.

In this study, we have introduced dummy variables to examine the effect of level of mother's education on the nutritional status of children.

Maxwell *et al.* (2000) and Ruel *et al.* (1998) argue that the effect of education is reflected through additional employment opportunities and income earning potential which lowers the significance of the education coefficient or make it insignificant, when income is included as one of the variables.

The evidence on role of father's education is not conclusive. Sahn (1990) and Alderman (1990) suggest that father's education is a proxy for income control and bargaining power within the household. Male preferences tend toward goods and services like entertainment, clothing, etc., which were less beneficial for children's nutrition in contrast to women's choices. This bias in preferences translated into a negative effect of father's education on nutritional status of children.

In our research work, the education level of father is introduced to examine its effect on nutritional status of children.

Woman's Empowerment

Woman's status is defined as woman's power relative to that of men in a household, community or region in which they live. Woman's participation in household decision making influences child nutrition through three major pathways: food security, caring practices for women and children, and health environment quality. Studies of Quisumbing and Maluccio (2003), Haddad *et al.* (1997) and Thomas (1997) have demonstrated that income or assets accruing to women or believed to be controlled by women are more likely than those of men to be allocated to expenditures that benefit children (for example, education), as well as themselves, such as food, clothing and health care. Smith *et al.* (2003) and Thomas (1997) find that women with low status tend to have weaker control over household resources, tighter time constraints, less access to information and health services, poorer mental health, and lower self-esteem which affect the kind of care which they give to their children and thus adversely affect the nutritional status of their children.

Hobcraft (2000), Leslie (1998) and McGuire and Popkin (1990) demonstrate that the effects of improvements in women's status on the nutritional status of children is not always positive because women with higher status are more likely to enter the labour force which may reduce the time they spend in childcare or breastfeeding, and the substitute caretaker may not be as good as mother.

In this work, mother is assumed to be empowered if she takes decisions involving her health care.

Parents Living Together

Olaniyan (2002) has highlighted another factor: that is, whether husband and wife live together or not. Evidence from urban Nigeria found that if couple lives together, it means better social integration and better access to community resources and thus, a better nutritional status for children.

In this study, whether parents are living together or not have been captured through a dummy variable.

Nutritional Status of the Mother

Nutritional status of the mother is an extremely crucial factor as it operates right from the birth of the child. It has been found that countries with higher percentages of low birthweight infants generally have a higher percentage of women with low BMI and a higher percentage of underweight children (ACC/SCN, 2000).

Studies by Martorell *et al.* (1998) and WHO (1995) indicate that malnourished mothers tend to give birth to low birthweight babies who tend to remain underweight especially in the early years.

Engle *et al.* (1999) and Ramalingaswami *et al.* (1996) observed that malnourished woman might be less capable of breastfeeding successfully. Micronutrient deficiencies, especially iron deficiencies cause fatigue and may affect women's cognitive performance and therefore, their ability to adequately care for a young child (Beard, 2001).

In this study, the nutritional status of the mother has been measured by BMI of the mother.

Age of the Mother

The age of the mother is a proxy for her care taking abilities. It has been observed that too young mothers may not have enough experience to carry out the child rearing (Mishra *et al.*, 1999). However, in some studies mothers's age is not a significant variable (Sahn, 1990; Olaniyan, 2002).

In this study, we have introduced age and square of mother's age to observe its effect on nutritional status of children.

2.3.3 Household-Specific Factors

Household Economic Resources

A key determinant of malnutrition is low income or poverty (UNICEF, 1990). Thus, improvement in economic status translates into improved nutritional status of children (Attaniaso *et al.*, 2004; Block, 2002; Girma and Genebo, 2002; Duflo, 2000; Mishra *et al.*, 1999; Strauss and Thomas, 1992; Sahn, 1990; Ward and Sanders, 1980; World Bank, 1980).

But many studies indicate that relationship between income growth and nutritional status is not strong. The income coefficient may be insignificant in studies by Thomas *et al.* (1992), Melville *et al.* (1988), Horton (1986), Ryan *et al.* (1984) and Wolfe and Behrman (1982). In part, the insignificance may be on account of multicollinearity. Further, the measure of nutritional status reflects the outcome of inputs over a long period of time; it is certainly possible that household income may not reflect long-term effects on nutritional status.

Other indicators of economic status like size of land holding, provision of electricity, type of house, cattle owned, etc., have also been used in the literature. There is mixed evidence in case of these measures as well. For example, Strauss (1990), Horton (1986) and Desai *et al.* (1970) find a positive influence of the size of landholding on the nutritional status, while Victora *et al.* (1985) and Cervantes *et al.* (1981) report it to be insignificant.

In our study, we have used size of the land holding, type of house and provision of electricity in the house as the variables representing the economic status of the household.

Size and Composition of Household

Among the other household characteristics that affect the level of care received is the size and composition of the household. There is mixed evidence as far as issue of household size is concerned. Melville *et al.* (1988)

suggests a negative correlation between household size and nutritional status. However, Behrman and Wolfe (1984) show that there are economies of scale; therefore, children of larger family size have improved nutritional status. However, Sahn (1990) found no effect of household size on the nutritional status of the preschool aged children of Cote d'Ivoire.

The structure and composition of the household also determine the nutritional status of the children. It is generally believed that older siblings (six years and above) do not directly compete for nurturing time with younger children and provide some child care assistance which results in better nutritional status of the young child. Also, controlling for size, the greater the number of adult women, better the nutritional status of the young child. Maxwell *et al.* (2000) finds a significant negative association between housholds with more children between 0 and 4 years and their health status. Sahn (1990) found a positive effect of older siblings and female adults but no negative effect of the number of children less than five years on anthropometric status of young children. The explanation given for this is the greater value of expenditure per adult equivalent unit with increase in the number of children less than five years and thus, greater availability of food and non-food goods per child.

In our study, we have used size and composition of household to examine its effect on nutritional status of children. To observe the effect of the household composition, household is decomposed into three groups using age and sex information.

Head of Household

In this study, the role of the head of the family has been analysed through a dummy variable.

The gender of the head of the household also has important implications for nutritional status of a child. Kennedy and Cogill (1987) find that children living in households headed by women are better nourished. In contrast, Olaniyan (2002) finds that female-headed households are associated with lower child health status in rural Nigeria.

Availability of Water and Sanitation Facility

Of all infections affecting young children in developing countries, none is as important as diarrhoeal diseases (Chen and Scrimshaw, 1983).

Epidemiological data show that diarrhoeal diseases are more prevalent precisely at those ages at which growth is most retarded. Diarrhoea is more common in the first 3 years of life and the highest prevalence is reported from 6 to 18 months of life. According to World Health Organisation (2004), 88 per cent of diarrhoeal disease is attributed to unsafe water supply, inadequate sanitation and hygiene. Improved water supply and sanitation reduce diarrhoea morbidity by 21 per cent and 37.5 per cent respectively.

The main source of infection is poor sanitation and water facility, poor personal and environmental hygienic conditions. The young malnourished children are at greater risk of illness because of lower immunity to infections.

Infection is the more common cause of anaemia among the preschool children than poor dietary intake (Asobayire *et al.*, 2001; Brooker *et al.*, 1999; Stoltzfus *et al.*, 1997). Poor sanitation, unhygienic environments and infectious diseases often deplete the body's stores of vital nutrients such as iron (Bhargava *et al.*, 2003; Gopalan, *et al.* 2000; WHO/FAO, 1996). Iron intakes are not significant predictors of haemoglobin status, while hookworm loads are negatively associated with the haemoglobin status (Bhargava *et al.*, 2003).

Studies by Checkley *et al.* (2004), Esrey (1996) and Esrey *et al.* (1992) show the positive effect of improved sanitation and water facilities, and hygienic conditions on nutritional status of the individuals. Maxwell *et al.* (2000), and Behrman and Wolfe (1982) show access to community toilets improves the health status of the children.

However, Hebert (1985) showed that the effect of sanitary behaviour depends on the age of the children considered. Children from 18 to 36 months of age benefit most from their own and their parent's sanitary behaviour. Older children benefit from availability of resources for hygiene. Children under 18 months of age tend to be unaffected by any of the sanitation-related variables considered.

Jalan and Ravallion (2001) demonstrate the positive health gains for children under five from piped water in rural India. However, these gains are not found for children in poor families, particularly when the mother is poorly educated. Here education is a proxy for knowledge about how to ensure that water is safe to drink and how best to treat illness. A similar result is also obtained by Attanasio *et al.* (2004) for poor Colombian children living in small municipalities.

Further, Esrey *et al.* (1992), McJunkin (1982), Anderson (1981) and Henry (1981) show that benefits from improved water occurred only when sanitation is improved and only when optimal water is present. Better water source alone does not yield health benefits as found in Pitt and Rosenzwig (1985).

Hence, we include both provision of sanitation facilities, and source and quality of water in our study.

2.3.4 Village-Specific Factors

Access to health care infrastructure improves the nutritional status. Recent studies by Thomas *et al.* (1992) and Lavy *et al.* (1996) show that increasing provision of basic health services, that is, birth services, availability of drugs, and immunisation improves the nutritional status of the children considerably. It is not only the direct provision of care to individuals but better prenatal and also postnatal care of mothers that leads to better nutritional status of the children. Peabody *et al.* (1998) show that Jamaican women with access to high quality prenatal care have higher birth weights than women with access to poor quality care. Barber and Gertler (2001) and Peabody *et al.* (1998) conclude that children who live in communities with high quality care are healthier.

Distance to the medical services or health infrastructure has no consistent result. Strauss (1990) showed that distance to health facilities is orthogonal to the anthropometric status of children in rural Cote d'Ivoire, while Barrera (1990) showed the expected inverse relationship in case of Philippines.

We examine the effect of accessibility to health facilities and sewerage system of the villages on the nutritional status of children in Indian context.

This review of literature suggests that the basic framework outlined in Chapter 1 with nutritional status (anthropometric outcome) as the output of a production function which has as its inputs-nutrient intake and non-nutrient inputs is appropriate. These non-nutrient variables can also be grouped as individual, parent, household and village specific variables.

3 Database

The two principal sources of data used in this study are the quinquennial surveys on consumer expenditure conducted by the National Sample Survey Organisation (NSSO) and National Family Health Survey (NFHS–2) coordinated by the International Institute of Population Sciences.[1] Both surveys are rich, nationally representative databases covering different aspects of households living in India. Since the present study pertains only to rural India, only the rural components of these data sources are used here. In the sections below, we introduce the two data sets in detail and highlight the important aspects used in our study.

3.1 Consumer Expenditure Surveys

The principal data source for this study is the NSSO's consumer expenditure surveys conducted once every five years. Unit record data for two years, corresponding to the survey periods January-December 1983 (the 38th round) and July 1999 to June 2000 (the 55th round) form the basis of the analysis. Our sample thus consists of nearly 77,000 rural households in 1983 and 70,000 rural households in 1999-2000.

A stratified two-stage sampling design was adopted by the NSSO, with census villages as the first stage units (FSU) and households being the second stage. In the rural sector, the sampling frame was provided by the 1981 and 1991 census list of villages. Each state/union territory (UT) was divided into one or more agroeconomic regions by grouping contiguous districts which are similar with respect to population density and cropping pattern. Within each region, each district normally formed a separate stratum. However, if size of the district exceeded two million, the district was split into two or more strata by grouping contiguous *tehsils*.

1. ORC Macro International, Calverton, Maryland, USA and the East-West Center, USA, provided technical guidance for NFHS-2.

Selection of the sample villages was done circular systematically with probability proportional to the population size. Further, the large villages were divided into hamlet groups having equal population content. Two hamlet groups were selected from the larger villages.

While listing the households in the selected villages, certain relatively affluent households were identified[2] and considered as second stage stratum 1 and the rest as second stage stratum 2. A total of 12 households were surveyed from the selected village, 2 from the first category and the rest from the second. Further, in the second stage stratum 2, the households are arranged according to the 'means of livelihood'. The means of livelihood were identified on the basis of major source of income as: (1) households self-employed in agriculture, (2) rural labour households and (3) others. The land possessed by the households was also ascertained and frame for selection was arranged on the basis of this information. The households were selected circular systematically from both the second stage strata.

The survey collects information on consumption and expenditure relating to a large number of food and non-food items, along with other household information including social group, education level and the age-sex composition of the household. Using a reference period of the last 30 days preceding the date of inquiry, it collects detailed consumption data in value and quantity terms. In all, the NSSO canvassed information on approximately 160 food items in 1983 and 140 food items in 1999-2000.

The survey is conducted in four sub-rounds over the course of the year, each corresponding to a period of three months. Equal number of villages was allotted for each of these sub-rounds. These four sub-rounds capture adequately the seasonal variations in India which affect the cropping pattern and thus, the availability of food in rural India. This information is utilised to address questions related to seasonality in nutrient intakes.

Rich though this source of data is, it is important to recognise that the unit of observation in the NSSO survey is the household. Intake figures are not separately available for members within the household; this implies that intra-household allocation issues cannot be addressed directly. However, in our exercise, we formulate a way that takes into account demographic

2. This was done for the 1999-2000 round to give due representation to the affluent and non-affluent classes as compared to the 1983 round.

composition in calculating household specific norm for the nutrient as discussed in section 4.2 and this has been used to compute prevalence of nutritional deficiencies in rural India.

3.1.1 The Comparability of the 55th and 38th Rounds

One change in the survey instruments used in the 55th round was the use of two recall periods. The NSS 55th round simultaneously collected information about the household's consumption both in the last 7 and in the last 30 days, in contrast to the uniform 30-day recall period in earlier rounds. It has been suggested that the use of a multiplicity of reference periods within the same round could have engendered confusion among the respondents and 'contaminated' the data, and further, that this would influence comparisons between the two survey rounds.

As far as poverty is concerned, the extent to which this methodological change affects poverty comparisons has been the subject of debate. This debate has been joined by several, for example, by Datt *et al.* (2003), Deaton (2001; 2003a; 2003b), Deaton and Drèze (2002), Sen (2000), Sundaram and Tendulkar (2002; 2003), Tarozzi (2004) and Visaria (2000). These studies conclude that there has been a less rapid decline of poverty at the all India level than has been suggested by the data, as a consequence of this change in methodology.

As far as food items are concerned, Chandrasekhar and Ghosh (2003) suggest that consumption expenditure, including that of food, would have been overstated in 1999-2000 as a consequence of this change. However, there is other evidence that the magnitudes of food intake are left uncontaminated. For instance, Sundaram and Tendulkar (2003) show that aggregate food intakes, canvassed separately in an abridged employment–unemployment module (which did not have a mixed reference period), are of comparable orders of magnitude to that in the consumer expenditure module. If at all, abridgement should have resulted in understating of consumption figures.

To deal with this issue, we compare consumption estimates of 55th round with that in the subsequent 56th and 57th rounds where a uniform recall period is used and see if there is any evidence of contamination in the 55th round. The premise is that food eating habits are unlikely to change dramatically within a year or so, thus, if there are differences in consumption between the 55th round on the one hand, and the 56th and 57th rounds on the other, these may be attributed to such contamination.

As indicated in Table 3.1, there are only slight differences in the average per capita per month food intake of major cereals in 55th, 56th and 57th rounds.

Table 3.1

Average Per Capita Per Month Consumption of Cereals in Rural India, 55th, 56th and 57th Rounds

(Kilograms Per Capita Per Month)

Monthly per capita consumption of	*55th round (1999-2000)*	*56th round (2000-01)*	*57th round (2001-02)*
Cereal	12.72	12.43	12.15
Rice	6.78	6.7	6.77
Wheat	4.55	4.59	4.12
Jowar	0.50	0.39	0.44
Bajra	0.38	0.33	0.36
Maize	0.32	024	0.30
Other cereals	0.18	0.17	0.16

Source: NSS 55th, 56th and 57th round reports.

This is broadly true also for the distribution of per capita expenditure spent over the major food items (Table 3.2). Cereals account for 22 per cent

Table 3.2

Percentage Distribution of Food Expenditures Across Major Food Groups, 55th, 56th and 57th Rounds

Food Item	*55th round (1999-2000)*	*56th round (2000-01)*	*57th round (2001-02)*
Cereals	22.2	20.0	19.2
Gram	0.2	0.1	0.1
Cereal substitutes	0.1	0.1	0.1
Pulses and its products	3.8	3.4	3.4
Milk and its products	8.8	8.7	8.4
Edible oil	3.7	3.4	3.7
Egg, fish, meat	3.3	3.6	3.4
Vegetables	6.2	5.9	6.6
Fruits	1.7	1.8	1.6
Sugar	2.4	2.4	2.2
Spices	3.0	2.3	2.4
Beverages	4.2	4.5	4.4
Total food	59.6	56.2	55.5

Source: NSS 55th, 56th and 57th round reports

of all food expenditures in the 55th round as compared to 20 per cent in the 56th and 19 per cent in the 57th rounds.

These results thus suggest that neither the average quantity of consumption nor the shares of different food items calculated for 55th round are out of line with 56th or 57th round results. Therefore, it is safe to assume that 38th and 55th rounds data are comparable at least as far as consumption of food items are concerned. Questions of comparability appear to matter more for poverty estimates.

3.2 Deriving Nutrient Intakes using Food Composition Tables

The NSS unit record data report information on food intakes—these must be converted to the equivalent amounts of macro and micronutrients. To convert the quantity of each of the food items canvassed in the 1983 and 1999-2000 to nutrient intakes (micronutrients and macronutrients), food composition tables taken from Nutritive Value of Indian Foods (Gopalan *et al.*, 2000) have been used. Thus, for each of the 160 food items in the 38th round and the 140 food commodities in the 55th round, the quantity consumed was multiplied by its nutrient content to derive the nutrient intake by the household. This was done for each of the nine nutrients considered in the study.

Aggregating across commodities provides an estimate of the total intake of that nutrient. For example, 100 gms of wheat contains 11.8 gms proteins, 1.5 gms fat, 346 kcal energy, 4.9 mg iron, 64 μg (micrograms) carotene, 0.45 mg thiamine, 0.17 mg riboflavin and 5.5 mg niacin (Gopalan *et al.*, 2000). For some of the items like 'other milk products', 'other leafy vegetables', 'other vegetables', 'other fresh fruits', and so on, we have used the closest possible food item or averaged out to get the nutrient content as these do not represent a single food item. For one of the survey years, the NSS also provided data on energy intakes by the household—this served as a check on the conversion factors used.

Also in some cases, consumption is reported only in value but not in quantity terms. For such commodities, we derived a nutrient content per rupee using appropriate price indices. For example, in case of 'other vegetables', NSS data are reported in rupee terms. We, therefore, compute the average nutrient content of the constituent vegetables, *viz.*, ash gourd, drumsticks, sem beans, cluster beans, *ghosala*, *karonda* and *tinda* in per kilogram terms. To get a rupee equivalent, we divide the derived nutrient content by an assumed price per kilogram of these vegetables.

It is important to note at the outset that these are slightly different from those in the published reports of the NSS. This is because of the commodity coverage which varied slightly in the various NSS rounds. While calculating the total intake of different nutrients per consumer unit per day, the NSS has excluded intoxicants group from 38th round and included for 55th round. To maintain the consistency in our analysis, we have excluded *pan*, tobacco and intoxicant groups from both the rounds.

There are, of course, limitations involved in this method. For example, it is well known that the nutritive value of a food item is sensitive to choice of cooking methods the range of which is ignored. Nor it is an indication of the amount of the nutrient that is bioavailable or absorbed by the body. Nevertheless, it is a relatively inexpensive way of obtaining not just the average intake but also its distribution.

3.3 The National Family Health Survey (NFHS-2)

The other principal source of data used in this study is the NFHS-2 conducted in 1998-99. The survey canvassed information on nutritional status, health and health care, fertility, mortality, and family planning.

Like the NSSO survey design, these surveys also use a stratified sample design. Thus, in each state, the rural sample was selected in two stages: at the first stage, the primary sampling units (PSUs), which are villages, are selected with probability proportional to population size (PPS). In rural areas, the 1991 census list of villages served as the sampling frame. Large villages (with more than a specified number of households, usually 500) were segmented, and two segments were selected randomly using PPS. In the second stage, the households to be interviewed were selected with equal probability using systematic sampling.

The survey collected information from 2,531 villages in 25 Indian states[3] from more than 65,000 ever-married women aged 15–49 years in

3. The survey excluded Tripura because of problems in collecting data.

rural India. The enumerators also collected detailed information for more than 18,000 children under the age of three years with respect to nutritional status, especially anthropometric measures (height and weight), and anemic status of the last two births since 1995-96 from these eligible women (NFHS–2).

NFHS-2 administered three types of questionnaires: the household questionnaire, the women's questionnaire and the village questionnaire.

The household questionnaire sought information on the demographic composition, including age, sex, marital status, relationship to the head of the household, education and occupation. It also collected information on the prevalence of asthma, tuberculosis, malaria and jaundice, and on health care seeking behaviour. Also collected were indicators of sanitation, type of housing, and ownership of land and other assets.

The woman's questionnaire elicited responses on gender roles and the treatment of women within the household. Further, information was collected on breastfeeding, feeding practices and recent occurrences of diarrhoea, fever and cough for young children.

In addition, the health investigator on each survey team measured the height and weight of each woman and each of her children born since January 1995 (in states where fieldwork started in 1998) or January 1996 (in states where fieldwork started in 1999). These data are used to calculate the three summary indices: weight-for-age, height-for-age and weight-for-height. These indices are expressed in standard deviations units (z-score) from the median for an international reference population.[4] Children who are more than two standard deviations below the reference median on any of the indices are considered to be undernourished, and children who fall more than three standard deviations below the reference median are considered to be severely undernourished.

The two main anthropometric indicators available for adults are height and weight. The reference median weight for adults varies among populations; the cut-off height below which a woman is considered

4. Based on the conclusion that growth potential up to age five does not differ across ethnic groups, the WHO (1995) recommends the use of a single global reference population for calculating anthropometric statistics for children under five. This has led to a systematic collection of standardised anthropometric data on a global basis, based on the National Center for Health Statistics/WHO reference population.

nutritionally deficient ranges between 140-150 cm. The body mass index (BMI) is defined as weight in kilograms divided by the height in metres squared (kg/m^2) and is used to indicate both thinness and obesity. Chronic energy deficiency (CED) is usually indicated when an individual has BMI less than 18.5. In our study, we have chosen BMI which is based on both height and weight to represent the anthropometric status of an individual and not height alone as discussed in section 2.3. Enumerators also took blood samples from each woman and her young children to assess prevalence rates of anaemia among women and children. An individual is said to be anaemic if haemoglobin level is below 12 gms per decilitre in case of women and below 11 gms per decilitre in case of children under age three years.[5]

At each village, a short, open-ended questionnaire was administered to the village head with questions on perceptions of major problems of the village and possible solutions. It also collected information on the availability of various facilities in the village (especially health and education facilities) and amenities such as electricity and telephone connections. For some of the regressions estimated in Chapter 6, the number of observations exceeds 18,000.

3.4 Merging of NSS and NFHS Data Sets

Both the NSS and the NFHS are, therefore, rich sources of data, canvassed at about the same time (1999-2000 for the 55th round of the NSS and 1998-99 for the second NFHS survey). Together these constitute a comprehensive database on socioeconomic status, dietary intakes and nutritional status. From NSS data (1999-2000), we get a detailed account of nutritional intakes of the households by applying nutrient conversions (Gopalan *et al.*, 2000) for the different food items consumed over the past 30 days. However, NSS gives no information with regard to nutritional status or incidence of diseases, morbidity or mortality estimates for the households.

While the NFHS-2 (1998-99) data is a nationally representative survey that provides detailed information on demographic and health parameters, it does not provide any information on household income and nutrient

5. Adjustment has been made for pregnant women, altitude of the place, smoking, etc.

intakes as it canvasses only limited information on food intakes (largely on food frequency—daily, weekly or never). Similarly, the number of food items canvassed for children under the age of three years extends only to consumption of mushy food, green leafy vegetables and fruits besides milk (breastfeeding as well as other milk).

To explore the relationship between nutritional status on one hand and nutrient intakes, socioeconomic and environmental variables on the other, the near-coincidence of the NSS survey in 1999-2000 and the NFHS survey in 1998-99 has been exploited to merge two data sets. Since the sets of households canvassed in the two data sets are different, these cannot be merged at the household level.

The merging is effected instead at the regional level. In each of these data sets, each state/UT is divided into one or more agroeconomic regions by grouping contiguous districts which are similar with respect to population density and crop pattern. Therefore, using the unit record data for each data set, a regional average of each of the variable is constructed. The total sample size is thus 63 regions, substantially more than if state-level averages had been used.

3.5 Nutrients and their Functions

It seems appropriate here to provide a brief description of the various nutrients and their functions in the human body.

Nutrients are organic and inorganic complexes contained in food, each with specific functions. Most natural food contains more than one nutrient. Nutritionists have categorised nutrients into macronutrients and micronutrients depending on the quantity of these required by the body (Park, 1997).

Macronutrients: These are proteins, fats and carbohydrates which are often called 'proximate principles' because they form the bulk of food.

Micronutrients: These are vitamins and minerals. These are required in small amounts which may vary from micrograms to several milligrams per day; micronutrients cannot typically be manufactured by the body. Therefore, they must be part of the diet or taken as supplements. A deficiency of even a small magnitude may contribute to learning disability, impair work capacity and illness.

A balanced diet is defined as one which contains a variety of food in the quantity and proportion such that the biological requirements of energy, proteins, fats, minerals and other elements are adequately met for maintaining health and well-being. It may also enable a person to withstand short periods of dietary stress. Nutritionists have increasingly recognised that a balanced diet is critical in preventing nutritional deficiencies.

The type and quantity of various foods that constitute the typical diet are based on sociocultural norms as well as economic considerations. For example, North Indian diets are wheat based, while south Indian diets have rice as the primary staple. Similarly, the poor tend to rely more on the so-called starchy staples, the cheapest sources of calories, while the rich have more diversified diets.

3.5.1 Calories

The total energy requirement is made up of two main components. The first is basal or resting energy. The amount of energy expended when the body is at complete rest (both mentally and physically) is termed as basal metabolism rate (BMR). The second component is the energy required for actual physical activity and thus, depends on the type of occupation the individual is engaged in. Energy is measured in calorie (kcal).[6] There are three components of food which provide this energy—carbohydrates, fats and proteins. In Indian diets, nearly 80 per cent of energy comes from carbohydrates, 9-10 per cent from protein and rest from fat (Gopalan *et al.*, 2000: 8). Thus, cereals form the chief source of energy in India.

The energy requirement of an adult man is 2,400 kcal per day. The requirement is lower for an adult woman.

3.5.2 Proteins

These are structural or bodybuilding materials of human life. They are essential in ensuring physical growth and development, for tissue maintenance and repair, and for healing and recovery from disease. The

6. Calorie is the amount of heat necessary to raise the temperature of one kg of water by 1°C from 14.5°C to 15.5° C.

amount of protein to be consumed to meet this requirement of body depends on the quality of dietary protein; the higher the quality, lower the requirement. The quality of protein depends on the pattern of amino acids it supplies[7]—the best quality protein is that which produces essential amino acids in a pattern similar to that of tissue proteins. Egg protein and human milk protein satisfy this criterion and are classified as the best quality protein and therefore, serve as the reference in defining the quality of other proteins. It is generally seen that animal proteins are of higher biological value than proteins from plant foods. Cereals contain 6-12 per cent protein but are generally deficient in lysine.

However, when eaten with pulses which are rich in lysine, the quality of protein is enhanced. A combination of cereal and pulses in the ratio of 5:1 has been found to be optimum combination in terms of supplying essential amino acids (Gopalan *et al.*, 2000: 27).

The adult requirement of egg protein is 0.7 g per kilogram of body weight, and 1 g per kilogram in terms of mixed vegetable protein. It needs to be emphasised that figures for protein requirement are valid only when other nutrients, particularly calories, in the diet are adequate.

3.5.3 Fat

Fats serve a number of functions in the body. They are a concentrated source of energy and are also important for absorption of fat-soluble vitamins such as carotene. Further, they are a source of essential fatty acids which have vitamin-like functions in the body.

Fats are of two kinds: visible and invisible. Visible fats, also termed added fats, are derived from both animal fat—butter and ghee—which are solid fats, or from vegetable fats—oils such as groundnut, mustard—which are liquid fats. Apart from visible fats, some amount of fat is also present in other food items such as cereals, pulses, oilseeds, milk, egg, meat, etc.

The minimal requirement of visible fat to meet essential fatty acid requirement is 15-25 g/day for different physiological groups; the essential fatty acid (EFA) requirement in turn has been placed at 3-6 per cent of total

7. The dietary proteins are broken down into simplest form called amino acids which can be absorbed by the body. These amino acids are used by the body to synthesise the protein needed by the body for various functions such as tissue building, formation of hormones, enzymes, etc.

energy intake depending upon age and physiological state. The invisible fat present in the diet is estimated to contribute to about 6 per cent of energy (Gopalan *et al.*, 2000: 6-7). Although the quantity of fat should be included in a well balanced diet but unlike proteins, it is not known with any degree of certainty. It is opined the upper limit of fat in the diet should not exceed 30 per cent of calories.

3.5.4 Iron

Iron is of great importance in human nutrition. The central function of iron is oxygen transport and cell respiration. It is also necessary for many other functions in the body: for example, the formation of haemoglobin, brain development and function, regulation of body temperature, and muscle activity. Rich sources of iron are cereals, millets, pulses and green leafy vegetables. Of the cereals, millets, *ragi* and *bajra* are very good sources of iron. Milk, a good source of several micronutrients, is a poor source of iron.

The adult body contains between 3-4 gm of iron of which about 60-70 per cent is present in the blood as circulating iron and the rest as stored iron in the spleen and liver. Most of the iron in the body is reutilised. Therefore, the amount of iron to be absorbed from daily diet is quite small and is approximately 1-3 mg depending upon age, physiological status and level of daily physical activity. Because of the body's limited capacity to absorb dietary iron, intakes need to be between 10-25 times the required iron (Gopalan *et al.*, 2000: 19).

The absorption of iron in the food, termed bioavailability, depends on a number of factors. The body tightly regulates the iron metabolism and an individual absorption of dietary iron is inversely related to one's iron status; there is greater absorption if there is low iron status. In addition, the form of iron influences the amount absorbed.

There are two forms of iron—heme and non-heme. The iron in animal sources (meat, fish, poultry) is about 40 per cent heme and 60 per cent non-heme (Carpenter and Mahoney, 1992; Monsen *et al.*, 1978). Non-heme iron is the iron in all plant food sources and in about 60 per cent of the animal food sources. About 25-35 per cent of heme iron is absorbed, while the absorption from non-heme iron varies between 3-8 per cent, depending on dietary factors as well as individuals' iron status (Bhargava *et al.*, 2001; Tseng *et al.*, 1997; Carpenter and Mahoney, 1992). Bhargava *et al.* (2001) extended algorithms given by Tseng *et al.* (1997) for calculating bioavailable iron from mixed diets, under the assumption that iron body stores were 0, 250 and 500 mg. For example, assuming body iron stores were 500 mg, the iron bioavailability (FEBIO) can be calculated as:

FEBIO (500) = 23*40% (FEMFP) + [3+8.93 log{(EF+100)/100}]*CT [FETOT-0.4 FEMFP]/100

where FEMFP is iron from meat, fish and poultry, EF is enhancing factor, CT is correction factor, FETOT is total intake of iron. And

(1) CT = -0.2869 ln_{10}(PHY)+ 0.1295, where PHY=mg of phytates in the meal.

(2) EF = (M + F + P) + AA, where meat (M), fish (F), poultry (P) are grams of animal tissue. AA is milligrams of ascorbic acid.

So the equation shows that iron absorption is enhanced with simultaneous intake of vitamin C and of heme iron, that is, a diet rich in vegetables, fruits and animal products. In contrast, dietary factors that inhibit the absorption of iron include carbonates, oxalates, phosphates and phytates found in whole grains, legumes, tea, coffee and certain vegetables. There is recent evidence that interaction of other nutrient affects iron absorption and utilisation. Vitamin A plays a role in the mobilisation of body iron stores. Poor vitamin A status is associated with iron deficiency. High intake of calcium inhibits the absorption of both heme and non-heme iron, and riboflavin deficiency tends to co-exist and interact with iron deficiency (Schultink and Gross, 1996; Gopalan *et al.*, 2000; Gross *et al.*, 2000).

Diets predominantly based on cereals permit only a low level of absorption in the range of 2-5 per cent, while diets containing relatively high levels of meat and fish permit 10-20 per cent absorption. Given that diets in India are cereal based, with low levels of consumption of meats, dietary intakes of iron need to be around 28 mg per day for an adult male (Gopalan, *et al.*, 2000). In general, women require more iron than men on account of losses during menstruation. Thus, more than the quantum of dietary iron intake, it is its bioavailability that is critical in determining nutrient sufficiency.

3.5.5 Vitamins

Vitamins are organic substances present in small amount in many foods. Vitamins are of two types: water-soluble (for example, vitamin B and vitamin C) and fat-soluble (vitamin A). Water-soluble vitamins are not accumulated in the body but are readily excreted, while fat-soluble vitamins are stored in the body. For this reason, excessive intakes of fat-soluble vitamins can prove to be toxic.

(a) Vitamin A

There are two forms of vitamin A found in food—retinol (pre-formed A) which is only in animal products such as egg yolk, liver, fish, butter, ghee, whole milk, curd; and carotene (pro-vitamin A) found in vegetable foods.

Among several types of carotenoids, β-carotene is the most important. The latter form is plant based and present in yellow, orange and green fruits and vegetables especially spinach, carrot, papaya. Carotenoids[8] are converted into vitamin A in the body. Carotene is, therefore, termed as pro-vitamin A. There are efficiency losses both in conversion and utilisation of pro-vitamins. Thus, 1 μg of carotene yields 0.5 μg of retinol, and of this only 50 per cent is absorbed. Therefore, taking into account the physiological conversion and absorption of β-carotene, 1 μg of β-carotene yields only 0.25 μg of retinol. Thus, the requirement of carotene is four times that of requirement retinol.[9] The daily requirement of vitamin A for an adult is estimated to be 600 μg of vitamin A or 2,400 μg of β-carotene.

Vitamin A is somewhat less stable than carotene. Light and atmospheric oxygen destroy vitamin A; similarly, prolonged heating causes destruction of vitamin A. Thus, green vegetables should be consumed fresh to get maximum vitamin A.

8. Since these pigments were isolated from carrot, they are called carotenes.
9. 1 μg β-carotene =0.25 μg retinol. If the diet contains both retinol and carotene, its vitamin A content can be expressed as: Retinol content (μg)= (μg) retinol+ (μg) β-carotene* (0.25)

Fat, protein, zinc and vitamin E assist the body in the absorption of vitamin A. Fat, in particular, is needed in the diet for maximum absorption. Because vitamin A is fat-soluble, the body is able to store up to six months supply of vitamin A (Gopalan *et al.*, 2000: 11-13).

(b) Vitamin B

There are several B-vitamins—of these, we include the most important, that is, thiamine, riboflavin and niacin. B-vitamins are essential for metabolism and utilisation of proteins, fats and carbohydrates in the body.

Thiamine

One of the main functions of thiamine is the utilisation of carbohydrates. In the absence of adequate amount of thiamine, full utilisation of sugar and starches for meeting energy needs is adversely affected. Its deficiency causes beri-beri. The need for thiamine increases when the proportion of carbohydrates is high. Or conversely, presence of fat in the diet decreases the need for this vitamin and hence, fat is said to be thiamine-sparing action.

Its requirements are closely related to energy intake and hence, are expressed in terms of energy intake, that is, about 0.5-2 mg per thousand kcal per day depending upon age, physiological status and the level of daily physical activity. The recommended dietary allowance (RDA) used here is 1.2 mg per day (Gopalan *et al.*, 2000: 15).

Thiamine occurs in all natural foods, although in small amounts. Important sources are whole wheat, rice, gram, yeast, pulse and oilseeds, especially groundnut. Meat, egg, fish, vegetables and fruits are not as rich sources of this nutrient. The main source of thiamine in the diet of Indian people is cereals (rice, wheat) which contribute to 60-85 per cent of total supply.

Riboflavin

Riboflavin is essential for metabolism and proper utilisation of proteins, fats and carbohydrates in the body. It is also essential for normal functioning of skin, intestinal and nervous system. It plays a fundamental role in cellular oxidation. It is a part of certain enzymes involved with energy metabolism.

Its daily safe requirement ranges from 0.7 to 2.2 mg per thousand kcal per day depending upon age, physiological status and the level of daily physical activity (Gopalan *et al.*, 2000: 16). We have used 1.4 mg per day as the RDA for riboflavin in the study.

Its deficiency causes soreness of tongue, cracking at the angles of the mouth, redness of the eye and burning sensation in the eyes. It also results in loss of psychomotor development in children. Recent studies indicate that common infection with respiratory infection can accentuate the deficiency of riboflavin.

Its richest sources are milk and its products, eggs, liver and green leafy vegetables. Cereals (whether whole or milled) and pulses are relatively a poor source but because of the bulk in which they are consumed, they contribute much of the riboflavin to Indian diets. Germination increases the riboflavin content of pulses and cereals.

Niacin (Nicotinic Acid)

It is essential for the metabolism of carbohydrates, proteins and fats. It is also necessary for the normal functioning of the skin, intestines and nervous system. Niacin is formed in the body from the amino acid—tryptophan which is present in all dietary proteins, and a part of which is converted into niacin. Food rich in niacin and/or tryptophan are liver, kidney, meat, fish legumes and groundnut.[10] The RDA is 6.6 mg per thousand kcal of energy intake. Lack of this vitamin in the diet leads to pellagra which is characterised by soreness of tongue, pigmented skin and diarrhoea.

(c) Vitamin C

It is a water-soluble vitamin. Of all the vitamins, it is the most sensitive to heat. Intake of vitamin C from fresh sources is necessary. It has an important role in tissue oxidation. It is needed for the formation of collagen which amounts to 25 per cent of total body protein. It helps in absorption of iron from vegetables. The main dietary sources of vitamin C are fresh fruit and green leafy vegetables. Traces of vitamin C occur in the fresh meat and fish but scarcely any in cereals. Germinating pulses contain good amounts as well. *Amla* is the richest source both in fresh and dry

10. Maize is a poor source of niacin as it occurs in the bound form unavailable to the consumer.

condition. Guava and chillies are cheap but rich source of vitamin C. The essential requirement for vitamin C is 40-60 mg per day. The cut-off used here is 40 mg per day (Gopalan *et al.*, 2000: 17).

3.6 Consequences of Nutritional Deficiencies

The consequences of malnutrition on community are direct and indirect. The direct effects are the occurrence of nutritional deficiencies such as protein-energy malnutrition—kwashiorkor and marasmus, vitamin and mineral deficiencies. The indirect effects are a high morbidity and mortality, retarded physical and mental growth and development, lowered vitality of people leading to lowered productivity, and reduced life expectancy. The high rate of maternal mortality, stillbirth and low birthweight are all associated with malnutrition.

In particular, xerophthalmia (dry eye) is the manifestation of vitamin A deficiency that is a widespread nutritional disorder leading to blindness in India.

Similarly, iron deficiency anaemia is a major nutritional problem in India particularly affecting women and children. It increases the risk of maternal and foetal mortality and morbidity. Conditions such as abortions, premature births and low birth weight are especially associated with low haemoglobin levels in pregnancy. Further, it impairs the cellular responses and immune functions and increases the susceptibility to infections. It also reduces the work performance and thus, lowers the efficiency which has great significance for the economy of the country.

Other significant causes of anaemia include nutritional deficiencies other than iron deficiency, genetic conditions, factors related to reproduction and infections that increase requirements for iron and other micronutrients. Malaria or helminthes infections are most common cause of anaemia in the developing world. These infections relate to problems of hygiene, sanitation, safe water and water management. Therefore, besides dietary improvements, other major areas of intervention relate improved water and sanitation facilities/practices and health care practices with regard to obstetric complications, particularly excessive bleeding, use of contraceptives that decrease blood loss, full immunisation of children, etc. (INACG, 2002).

The other common nutritional deficiencies observed are B-complex deficiencies. Riboflavin deficiency causes soreness of tongue, cracking of mouth, redness of eyes, burning sensation in eyes and scaliness of skin between nose and lips. Pellagra is caused by deficiency of niacin. It also causes soreness of tongue, pigmented skin and diarrhoea. Scurvy, a vitamin C deficiency, causes weakness, bleeding of gums and defective bone growth. However, it is not as common in India as other vitamin deficiencies. Prolonged deficiency of thiamine leads to the disease called beri-beri which results in loss of appetite, tingling and numbness in the legs and hands, palpitation, breathlessness, and weakening of heart muscles (Gopalan *et al.*, 2000).

4 Methodology

In Chapter 3, a detailed account of the unit record from two rich data sets NSS (1983, 1999-2000) and NFHS-2 (1998-99) has been discussed which gives us understanding about what information is available in terms of consumption pattern, socioeconomic variables and nutritional status indicators of rural Indian population.

In the present chapter, we take up the task of defining a methodology that has been used to compute nutrient intakes and assess these in terms of nutritional sufficiency criteria using the Foster-Greer-Thorbecke (FGT) class of indices as discussed in sections 4.1 and 4.2. Further, section 4.3 describes a method of estimation of nutrient demand functions which explore the role of various explanatory factors like income, occupational status, education, seasonality, etc., in determining the nutrient demand. The system of nine nutrient demand functions is estimated using seemingly unrelated regression (SUR) estimates.

Using the National Family Health Survey (NFHS-2) data, section 4.4.1 deals with methodology to study the determinants of nutritional status (standardised weight-for-age *z*-score for children under age three) using the fixed effect specification at the state, village, household and parent level. Section 4.4.2 explains the method which has been used to identify the relationship between regional level estimates of dietary-socioeconomic variables and nutritional status of children and mother obtained from merged National Sample Survey (NSS) and NFHS data sets.

4.1 The Recommended Dietary Allowance

In determining the adequacy or inadequacy of nutrient intakes, it is necessary to compare actual intakes with a norm. However, the choice of a norm can be particularly problematic. For energy, it is common to use a per capita norm based on a recommended daily allowance (RDA) of 2,400 kcal per capita per day. Yet, requirements vary by occupational status and location as well. Similarly, there are inter-individual and inter-ethnic variations in metabolism (Gopalan *et al.*, 2000; Svedberg, 2000).

In India, it is the Indian Council of Medical Research (ICMR) that is responsible for establishing the RDAs for energy and other nutrients. These RDAs are defined at a level at which 97.5 per cent of the individuals in the given group would meet their requirements.

These are set separately for each age group and by gender, and for pregnant and lactating women. For many nutrients, requirements also vary by activity status. For example, because of differences in life styles, the urban norm is set below the rural norm of 2,400 kcal per capita per day by 300 kcal per capita per day. Similarly, the energy requirements for adult males involved in non-mechanised farm in Tamil Nadu would be different from that of a highly mechanised farm in Punjab; this level of detail is, however, not taken into consideration. In general, over time, RDAs for energy have decreased in view of changing lifestyles that have become more sedentary.

Also taken into account are dietary patterns. For instance, it is known that proteins sourced in cereals are of lower quality than those from eggs or milk (section 3.5.2). The RDA for proteins thus takes into account the lower quality of proteins in the average Indian diet. Similarly, iron sourced in cereals is less bioavailable than that from meat sources, and the Indian RDA takes this into account and is, therefore, set at a level corresponding to five per cent bioavailability diet (Gopalan *et al.*, 2000).

Requirements also vary by climate. Energy expenditures are higher for populations living in extreme (hot, cold or high altitude) environments (Askew, 1995).

Adjustments may be required on account of extra energy needed to recover from frequent attacks or illness which may occur as a result, for example, of a poor living environment. As noted in Briscoe (1979), each degree of fever can increase the metabolic rate by as much as eight per cent. Thus, nutrient requirements can depend not just on personal characteristics but also on the quality of the living environment.

The use of an average weight and body mass index (BMI) on which to base the RDA has also been questioned. The basal metabolic rate (BMR) on which energy requirements are based, is in turn based on body weight. It has been argued that this reference weight differs between the poor and the rich, for the poor may face greater risk of economic shocks or seasonal vulnerability, and that there should be some allowance by way of an excess weight as buffer (Svedberg, 2002).

Thus, while construction of the RDA does attempt to take into account variations in age, sex and occupational status, it cannot incorporate the diversity in factors on which nutrient requirements depend. However, many micronutrient requirement distributions are relatively invariant to differences in the living environment. The intake of vitamin A, vitamin C and iron are based on growth requirements (in terms of age and gender) being independent of activity status, while daily allowances for vitamin B are related to energy intakes (Gopalan *et al.*, 2000).

Yet, another line of literature argues against the use of any fixed norm, as the human regulatory mechanism allows energy expenditure to adapt to changes in nutritional intake. This individual adaptability means that there are multiple intake equilibria at which body weight is locally maintained, although there are biological limits to adaptation. The possibilities of downward adaptation clearly become negligible at low intake levels (Payne, 1975; Sukhatme, 1982; Srinivasan, 1981, 1985; Seckler, 1982).

Also important to mention is the behavioural approach to norms, as exemplified by Minhas (1991). The idea is to determine energy intake levels at which consumers begin to feel food-rich—that is, the intake level at which households transition from being net recipients of food to net providers of food. These behaviourally derived norms vary significantly depending on culture, habits, spread of education, etc. They are much lower in states like Gujarat or Tamil Nadu than they are in Punjab or Haryana.

Note that although there is an extensive debate over the assessment of calorie requirement, norms associated with other nutrients have not received as much attention.

An important exception is a relatively new literature that has argued against the use of RDAs to determine the prevalence of inadequacy in a group of people. It is argued that by definition, the RDA is set at the level at which a large majority of people (97.5%) would have met their requirements. Since for most micronutrients, the distribution of intakes is independent of the distribution of the nutrient requirements, the use of RDA to determine the head count ratio of nutrient inadequacy might result in overestimation of its prevalence.

Instead, the recommendation is to use an estimated average requirement (EAR) of the nutrient, which corresponds to the median of the distribution of requirements for computing the head count ratios. The method is modified for iron, as the distribution of requirements is skewed largely on account of the fact that iron requirements of women are greater than men. Also, in case of energy, the distribution of intakes and requirements cannot be assumed to be independent, and the use of an estimated energy requirement (EER) is suggested.

It is only for assessing the probability of inadequacy at the individual level that RDAs continue to be used (Murphy *et al.*, 2002; Barr *et al.*, 2003). The Indian RDAs are set out in Table 4.1.

For this study, for reasons noted above, we continue to use an RDA based norm to evaluate the prevalence and extent of nutrient deficiency.

It is clear that the issue of an appropriate norm is a contentious one, and one on which there appears little consensus. Yet it provides a guide for nutritional surveillance and planning and is the reason we use it here.

4.2 Computing Nutrient Deprivation

In computing nutrient deprivation, the usual practice is to obtain estimates of per capita intakes and compare these with the RDAs outlined in Table 4.1. Instead, we exploit the demographic information available for each household to construct a household-specific norm rather than using a per capita norm. This overcomes the criticism that the aggregation implicit in computing per capita average intakes leads to the neglect of differences in requirements in age and gender. While this method cannot answer the other issues raised above, it does represent an improvement over the use of a per capita based norm. As demonstrated in Meenakshi and Vishwanathan (2001), the use of household-specific norm significantly alters the magnitude of head count ratios of insufficient intakes.

Table 4.1

Recommended Dietary Allowances of Various Nutrients for Indians

(Per Day)

Group	*Particulars*	*Calories (kcal)*	*Protein (gms)*	*Fat (gms)*	*Iron (gms)*	*Carotene (μg)*	*Thiamine (mg)*	*Riboflavin (mg)*	*Niacin (mg)*	*Vitamin C (gms)*
Men	Sedentary work	2425	60	40	28	2400	1.2	1.4	16	40
Women	Sedentary work	1875	50	40	30	2400	0.9	1.1	12	40
Infants	0-12 months	721	12.95	0	0	1200	0.3675	0.4275	4.76	25
Children	1-3 years	1240	22	45	12	1600	0.600	0.700	8	40
Children	4-6 years	1690	30	45	18	1600	0.9	1	11	40
Children	7-9 years	1950	41	46	26	2400	1	1.2	13	40
Boys	10-12 years	2190	54	42	34	2400	1.1	1.3	15	40
Boys	13-15 years	2450	70	42	41	2400	1.2	1.5	16	40
Boys	16-18 years	2640	78	42	50	2400	1.3	1.6	17	40
Girls	10-12 years	1970	57	42	19	2400	1	1.2	13	40
Girls	13-15 years	2060	65	42	28	2400	1	1.2	14	40
Girls	16-18 years	2060	63	42	30	2400	1	1.2	14	40

Source: Nutritive value of Indian Foods (Gopalan *et al.*, 2000)

Thus, for example, for energy, a household specific norm is defined as follows:

RDA (hhcal) = 2400 * man + 1875 * woman + 721 * infant + 1240 * child13 + 1690 * child46 + 1950 * child79 + 2190 * boy1012 + 1970 * girl1012 + 2450 * boy1315 + 2060 * girl1315 + 2640 * boy1618 + 2060 * girl1618

where man refers to the number of men 18 years and older; woman refers to the number of women 18 years and older; infant refers to children aged less than one year; child13 refers to children aged between 1 and 3; child46 refers to children aged 4 to 6 years; child79 refers to children aged 7 to 9 years; boy1012 and girl1012 refer to the number of boys and girls aged between 10 and 12 respectively; boy1315 and girl1315 refer to the number of boys and girls between 13 and 15 respectively; finally, boy1618 and girl1618 refer to the number of boys and girls between 16 and 18 years of age respectively.

Similarly, the household-specific RDAs for all other nutrients can be calculated by using the latest recommendations given by the Expert Committee constituted by Indian Council of Medical Research (ICMR) as in Table 4.1.

We have assumed the activity status to be sedentary, as no information is available regarding the occupational status of individual household members. This choice is natural for it corresponds most closely to the 2,400 kcal norm for calories that is commonly used in the Indian literature for people living in rural areas. This assumption about sedentary status is not critical as the RDAs for most of the other nutrients, especially protein, fat, iron, vitamin A and vitamin C, do not vary much by activity status as does the RDA for calories.

The nutrient intakes computed at the household level may be compared against the RDAs constructed at the household level to measure the inadequacy of nutrient intakes. To do this, we use the familiar FGT class of measures. While the FGT measures have been applied extensively in the poverty literature, their application to nutrient deficiency is relatively rare. Exceptions include Meenakshi and Vishwanathan (2001, 2003) and Jha (2003). Here we extend the application of the framework to include micronutrients for the first time in the literature.

The FGT measure (weighted)[1] is given by (Foster *et al.*, 1984):

$$FGT(\alpha) = \frac{1}{N}\sum_{i=1}^{q} w_i \left(\frac{Z_i - Y_i}{Z_i}\right)^{\alpha},$$

where Z_i is the nutrient norm for the ith household, Y_i is the ith household's nutrient intake, N is the total population (Σw_i), q is number of nutrient deprived households and w_i is the product of combined multiplier and household size.

The parameter, α, defines the type of nutrient deficiency measure. Thus, when $\alpha=0$, the *FGT* (0) index collapses to the familiar head count ratio of people with insufficient nutrient intakes, henceforth referred to as HCR. When $\alpha=1$, the index *FGT* (1) measures the average deficit or gap of nutrient with respect to the norm, weighted by the proportion of those who are thus deprived. When $\alpha=2$, the index *FGT* (2), square of the nutrient deficiency gap, measures the severity of nutrient deficiency, as it gives a higher weight to people whose intakes are far below the norm.

The RDAs of different nutrients considered here are used to calculate magnitude, depth and severity of the deprivation in terms of FGT class of indices (1984).

4.3 Nutrient Demand Functions

The measurement of nutrient deficiencies with the help of FGT indices provides a description of the magnitude, depth and severity of nutrient deficiencies and how these have changed over time, as detailed in Chapter 5. In Chapter 6, we examine various factors that influence demand for nutrients. It gives an insight to what role does income, occupational structure, social status, seasonality, education, head of the household, etc., play in determining demand for the nutrient intakes.

Following the work of Lancaster (1971), we work directly in the nutrient space rather than in the commodity space. Nutrient demand functions may be specified as functions of income, and demographic, socio-economic and other variables. Thus, we estimate a direct relationship

1. When weighted FGT index is used, it gives us the percentage of the total population which is deficient in the intake of a particular nutrient.

between nutrient intakes and the factors that determine them as detailed below. This approach has also been followed by Lancaster *et al.* (2004), Gibson and Rozelle (2002), Meenakshi and Vishwanathan (2001), Roy (2001), Subramanian and Deaton (1996), Behrman and Deolalikar (1987) and Behrman and Wolfe (1984). We estimate Engel functions for each of the nine nutrients as:

$$Y_{it} = f\,(X_t, Z_t)$$

where $i=1$ to 9 (calorie, protein, fat, thiamine, riboflavin, niacin, carotene, niacin and iron); t is for the tth household; Y is per capita nutrient intake; X is the monthly per capita expenditure and Z is the vector of other characteristics which includes occupational status of household, sub-rounds, household size and composition, education, social status and head of the household .

Per Capita Expenditure

Per capita expenditure is indicative of the purchasing power of the household. Income based interventions can be effective policy instruments to effect improvements in the nutrient intakes if income variables are significant. As noted in Chapter 2, the literature suggests that the income elasticity of energy demand may be high, although there are other studies which indicate that it is low (see section 2.2.1).

Occupational Status (Producer *versus* Non-producer Households)

The nature of employment has an important bearing on nutrient intakes independent of its effect through income, not only because the physical requirement of various nutrients depends on the kind of activity undertaken by workers as shown by Pitt (1983). Households involved in cultivation have access to agricultural products and therefore, can have higher consumption because of self-consumption or being paid in kind. This has been demonstrated in the context of calories in rural India by Subramanian and Deaton (1996) and Meenakshi and Vishwanathan (2001) who showed that self-employed agricultural households and agricultural labour households have higher calorie intake than other labour households.

We capture the effect of occupational status of the rural Indian household on nutrient intakes through introduction of four dummy variables—HHTYPE1, HHTYPE2, HHTYPE3, HHTYPE4 representing households self-employed in agriculture, self-employed in non-agriculture, other labour, and 'others' households respectively, and all the results are analysed with reference to the base category of agricultural labour households.

Seasonality

The seasonality in agricultural production may translate into seasonality in consumption in the absence of consumption smoothing. This in turn may be reflected in seasonality of nutrient intake in rural India, especially for those nutrients sourced in fruits and vegetables that are typically not stored. Seasonality has been included in studies by Meenakshi and Vishwanathan (2001), Bouis and Novenario-Reese (1997), Ravallion (1990) and Bouis and Haddad (1992). In the Indian context, Meenakshi and Vishwanathan (2001) suggest there is no significant seasonality in the calories and protein intake because of seasonality in production.

Exploiting the fact that the consumer expenditure surveys are conducted over four sub-rounds, we introduce three seasonal dummies in the nutrient demand functions as OD, JM, AJ representing October-December, January-March and April-June seasons, and analyse seasonality in nutrient intakes by testing the significance of these coefficients with reference to July-September as the base sub-round or season.

Household Size and Composition

The size and composition of a household may influence per capita intake of nutrients. Household size (HHSIZE) is included to account for the possible economies of scale which are widely reported in the literature. If there are economies of scale in consumption, this would imply larger households with the same level of income are better off than smaller households (Deaton and Paxson, 1998).

To understand the role of household size, we introduce logarithm of household size, ln (HHSIZE), as an explanatory variable. Studies such as Meenakshi and Vishwanathan (2001) and Subramanian and Deaton (1996) show that the coefficient for household size is negative for per capita intake of energy.[2] The negative sign indicates that per capita consumption of calories declines with increase in household size.

Household composition also influences per capita nutrient intakes: adults consume more than children do.[3] To capture the effect of household composition on per capita nutrient intake, we construct three dummy variables with respect to age and sex: proportion of adult females (PROADFE), proportion of male children (PROCHMALE) and proportion of female children (PROCHFE) in the household. The reference category is proportion of adult males in the household.

Social Status

In this research work, we introduce a dummy variable, SCST, taking a value 1 if it is a scheduled caste or scheduled tribe household and 0 otherwise, to understand whether these groups are actually more vulnerable to micronutrient deprivation compared to other households. In the case of energy, the work of Subramanian and Deaton (1996) and Meenakshi and Vishwanathan (2001) suggest that nutrient intake among the SC/ST are no different from those of other communities, once differences in income and other characteristics are taken into account.

Education

The effect of education, especially of women, on nutrient demand is well documented in the literature. The evidence appears to be mixed. For example, Roy (2001) and Pitt and Rosenzweig (1985) found education to be insignificant, while Bouis and Novenario-Reese (1997) reported an insignificant education coefficient for most of the nutrients considered. Behrman and Wolfe (1984), however, found that mother's schooling had a positive effect on nutrient intakes (see section 2.2.6).

In this study, we attempt to capture whether literacy has any significant impact on nutrient intakes by defining a dummy variable, EDUC, which takes value 1 if any adult member of the household is literate and 0 otherwise.

---

2. These formulations also include household composition variables.

3. We also include a gender disaggregation to account for possible differences in impact on nutrient intakes. While such a gender disaggregation has also been used to test indirectly for gender bias in the literature (see for example, Lancaster *et al.*, 2004; Roy, 2001 and Subramanian and Deaton, 1996), this is not the focus of this book.

Male *versus* Female-headed Households

In keeping with the literature, Meenakshi and Vishwanathan (2001) and Bouis and Novenario-Reese (1997) we introduce the role of the head of the family in determining the demand of nutrient intakes through a dummy variable, HEAD, which takes value 1 if headed by male and 0 otherwise. It is usually assumed that women are better informed about preparation and contents of food and thus, could better take care of nutritional status of the household.

We assume that prices are same for all households in particular year of the survey. Thus, price does not enter as a specific explanatory variable as in a usual demand function.[4] Therefore, we explain the nutrient demand in terms of income and other covariates as explained above and set out in Table 4.2.

Table 4.2

Correlates of Nutrient Intakes: Definitions of Explanatory Variables Used

Variable	*Definition*
MPCE	Log of monthly per capita total expenditure (Rs)
HHTYPE1	1 if household is self-employed in agriculture, 0 otherwise.
HHTYPE2	1 if household is self-employed in non-agriculture, 0 otherwise.
HHTYPE3	1 if household is other labour, 0 otherwise.
HHTYPE4	1 if household is 'others' household, 0 otherwise.
Base category	Agricultural labour households
OD	October-December
JM	January-March
AJ	April-June
Base season	July-September
Household size	1,2,3……(numerals)
PROADMALE	Proportion of adult males
PROADFE	Proportion of adult females
PROCHMALE	Proportion of male children
PROCHFE	Proportion of female children
Reference category	Proportion of adult males
SCST	1 if it is scheduled caste and scheduled tribe household, and 0 otherwise
EDUC	1 if any adult member of the household is literate, and 0 otherwise.
HEAD	1 if headed by male, and 0 otherwise.

4. For a small subset of the commodities in the NSS, it is not possible to compute unit values.

4.3.1 Method of Estimation

The fact that these nutrient intakes are derived from the consumption of same household food basket, suggests that these equations be estimated simultaneously. Further, the error terms in the nutrient demand function are likely to be correlated which gives rise to use of joint estimation technique, SUR estimation. At the same time, each nutrient demand function has the same right hand side variables. This implies that efficient set of estimates may be obtained by using a feasible generalised least squares estimator (Judge *et al.*, 1988).

For each state, these Engel functions are estimated in the computer package STATA using MYSUREG command along with SVYSET command which defines survey settings and weights to be used. Since the explanatory variable is in per capita terms, the weight is defined correspondingly as the household weight (combined multiplier) multiplied by household size.

4.3.2 The Choice of Functional Form

As widely discussed in the literature, non-linearities may characterise the relationship between nutrient intake and income because the poor are likely to have larger nutritional responses to income increases than the rich. This issue of non-linearity has been explored by Ravallion (1990), Strauss and Thomas (1990) and Subramanian and Deaton (1996) who conclude that elasticity is higher for poorer households. The work of Meenakshi and Ray (1999) suggests inclusion of quadratic income term as appropriate in Indian context. This has also been corroborated by Roy (2001) for Indian data.

To better understand the relationship between nutrient demand and income for all income levels, non-parametric regression may be an appropriate tool because it makes no assumption about functional form, allowing the data to 'speak for themselves' (Delgado and Robinson, 1992). However, non-parametric techniques suffer from what has been termed the 'curse of dimensionality' which makes multivariate estimation difficult; many non-parametric regressions are restricted to bivariate relationships.

In this research work, we use the advantage of non-parametric approach for determining correct specification of income term in the nutrient demand function. As most of the other variables are discrete, the question of functional form is not as important, and gains from using non-parametric regression are less apparent for the other variables besides income.

Method

We choose two states, Bihar and Punjab, representing the poorest and the richest state of rural India respectively to conduct this exercise for 1999-2000. This procedure involves three steps and takes advantage of the Frisch, Waugh and Lovell (FWL) theorem.

First, we estimate a system of nine nutrient demand function, excluding logarithmic value of monthly per capita income and including all the other factors as a set of explanatory variables using SUR. That is, we estimate $\ln Y_{it} = f_i(Z_t) + \varepsilon_{it}$ where, i is the nutrient, t is for the tth household, lnY is logarithm value of per capita nutrient intake, Z is the vector of other characteristics excluding income and ε_{it} is the error term, and obtain the predicted values of nutrient intakes.

Second, we obtain residuals by subtracting predicted value from the actual value of the nutrient intake. In other words, these residuals are reflective of the variation in nutrient intakes not explained by the set of variables other than income.

Third, we non-parametrically regress estimated residuals on logarithmic value of monthly per capita income using the KERNREG procedure in the computer package STATA.

The shape of the curve would depict the polynomial degree of the income term to be included in the nutrient demand function.

Result

Figures 4.1 and 4.2 depict the non-parametric relationship between logarithmic value of monthly per capita income and residuals saved for each of nine nutrients in states of Bihar and Punjab, representing the poorest and the richest state of India respectively. The shape of the non-parametric graphs suggests that the inclusion of quadratic term of logarithmic value of monthly per capita income in the parametric specification is appropriate. Since it is evident in all the nine nutrients for the set of both states considered, one could generalise this specification for other states and 1983 data set as well.

Figure 4.1

Punjab, Plot of Non-parametric Regression of Residuals from SUR on Logarithm of Per Capita Expenditure

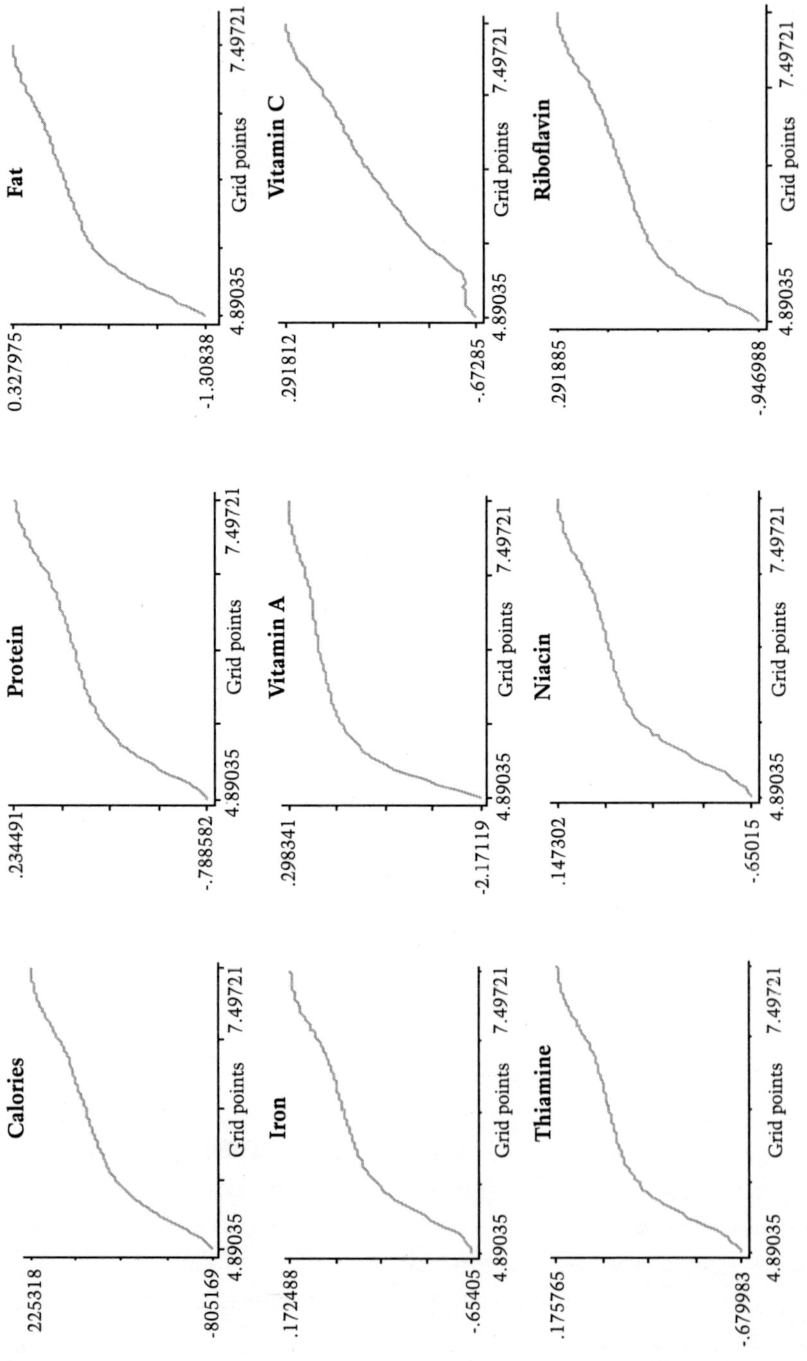

Figure 4.2

Bihar, Plot of Non-parametric Regression of Residuals from SUR on Logarithm of Per Capita Expenditure

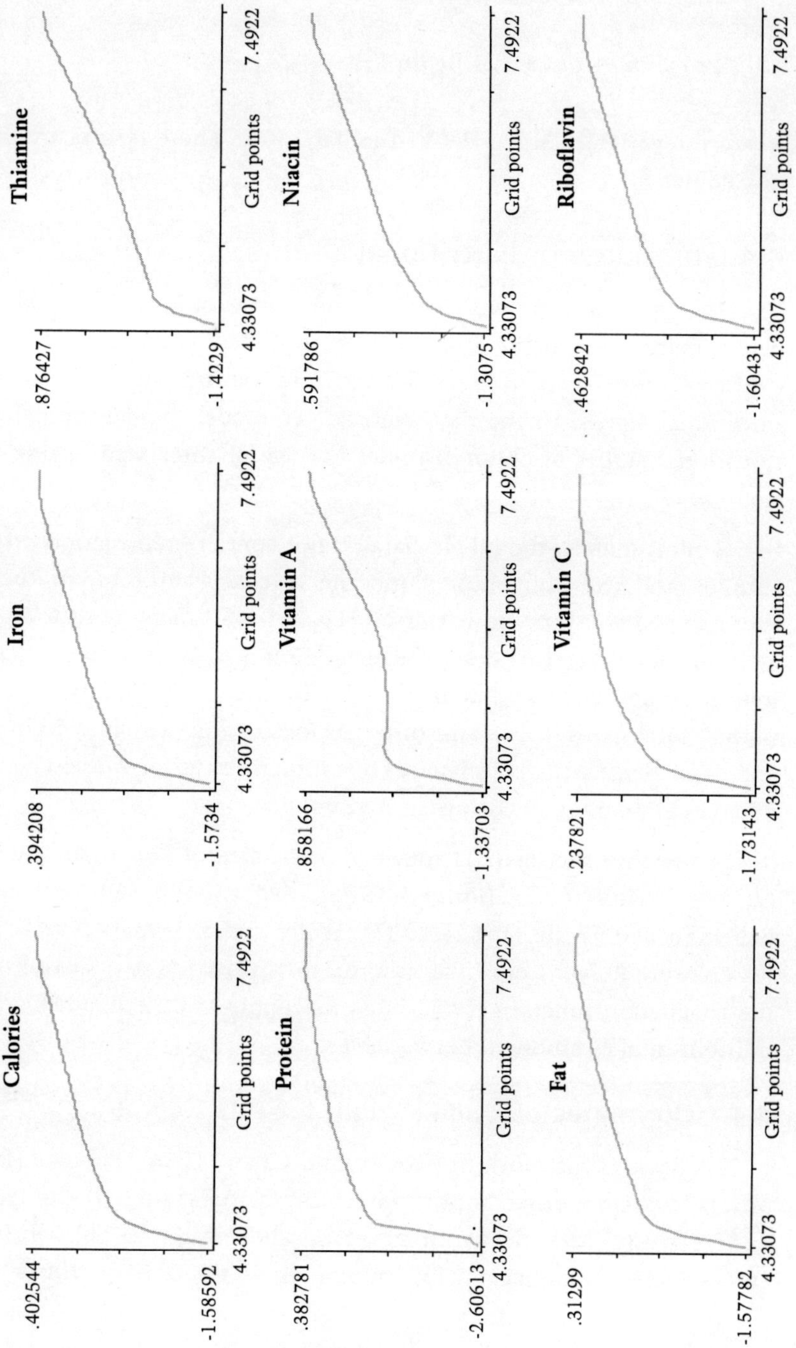

Therefore, the Engel function we estimate using SUR takes the form:

$$\ln Y_{it} = \alpha_i + \beta_{1i} \ln X_t + \beta_{2i} (\ln X_t)^2 + \beta_{3i} Z_t + \varepsilon_{it}$$

where the variables are as defined in Table 4.2. These results are discussed in Chapter 6.

4.4 Correlates of Nutritional Status

In this section, we discuss the methodology for studying the determinants of nutritional status of rural Indian population. Two separate exercises have been undertaken to understand the correlates of the nutritional status. In the first exercise, we model the determinants of the nutritional status of children under the age of three years using the data from NFHS-2.

Unfortunately, the NFHS data do not contain information on nutrient intakes and the household's income levels. Therefore, in the second exercise, we combine both the NFHS and NSS data sets for rural India at the regional level as described in section 3.4. We use nutritional status indicators and environmental variables from the NFHS data, and nutrient intake, total expenditure and other socioeconomic variables from the NSS data, and identify the correlates of nutritional status for women between 15-49 and children under the age of 3 years.

Following the basic framework of studies of Behrman and Skoufias (2004), Strauss and Thomas (1995), Alderman (1990), Sahn (1990), Behrman and Wolfe (1982; 1987), Wolfe and Behrman (1984), Pitt and Rosenzweig (1985), etc., we assume nutritional status is the output of the production function that has as its inputs—nutrient intakes and non-nutrient intakes among other variables.

4.4.1 Correlates of Child Weight for Age Scores

Following the work of Mosley and Chen (1984), Schultz (1984) and others, we categorise 'input' variables as individual (i), household (h) and village (v) level determinants. Household variables (h) can be further grouped into parent-specific (p) and household resource-specific (r) variables.

All these variables are estimated using the child, parent, household, village and state level fixed effects.

$$NS_{ihv} = f(X_i, X_h, X_v) + \varepsilon_{ihv}$$

where NS_{ihv} is the nutritional status of ith child living in the hth household and v^{th} village; and X_i, X_h, X_v are the individual, household and village level variables respectively. Household variables, X_h, have been classified into parent-specific, $X_{h(p)}$, and household resource-specific, $X_{h(r)}$, variables. ε represents unobserved characteristics.

Therefore, we have:

$$NS_{ihv} = f(X_i, X_{h(p)}, X_{h(r)}, X_v) + \varepsilon_{ihv}$$

(a) Specification of the Variables

Nutritional Status (NS)

Standardised weight-for-age *z*-score is used as an indicator of nutritional status of children under the age of three years as it is a measure of both acute as well as chronic undernourishment. This is a preferred measure also because the problems associated with the measurement of height are much more than weight as it requires proper position/posture of the body that may be more difficult to ensure for children under three as discussed in section 2.3.

The standardised weight-for-age *z*-score (NS_i) is given by National Center for Health Statistics (NCHS)/WHO,

$$NS_i = \frac{W_i - \mu_i}{\sigma_i}$$

where W_i is the observed weight of the child, μ_i is the reference median weight of child of that particular gender and age, and σ_i is the standard deviation of the reference population of that particular gender and age.

To make the interpretation in terms of changes in weight as compared to standardised weight-for-age *z*-score (NS_i), the following relationship can be used:

$$\frac{\partial NS_i}{\partial X} = \frac{\partial (W_i - \mu_i)/\sigma_i}{\partial X}$$

where X represents any of the right hand side variables. Assuming μ_i and σ_i are given for reference population of a particular gender and age, we get:

$$\frac{\partial W_i}{\partial X} = \sigma_i \frac{\partial (NS_i)}{\partial X}$$

In our research work, we have arbitrarily chosen underweight male child of age nine months to discuss the impact of various socioeconomic and dietary variables on his weight as well as change in standardised weight-for-age *z*-score. The value of sigma (σ_i) for this reference child is 0.96932.

Individual-specific Factors (X_i)

The individual-specific factors can be grouped into nutrient intakes and non-nutrient factors. The rationale for including these variables is detailed in section 2.3.

Nutrient Intakes

Since the NFHS data do not contain data on nutrient intakes, we use as proxies for nutrient intakes—the current breastfeeding status and frequency of complementary diet received in the form of solid mushy food, green leafy vegetables and fruits by the child in a household. Breastfeeding status is defined through dummy variable which takes a value 1 if the child is still being breastfed and 0 otherwise. Frequency of intakes of green leafy vegetables, fruits and other milk is represented through dummy variables—for 'daily' and 'sometimes' intake where 'never' is the reference category.

Non-nutritive Factors

The actual absorption or utilisation of nutrient intakes depends on the health of the child (Marotrell and Habicht, 1986 and other studies reviewed in section 2.3). To account for this, we use the health information on whether the child suffers from fever or diarrhoea in the past week. It is represented through a dummy variable which takes a value 1 if child had diarrhoea (or fever) and 0 otherwise.

Among the demographic factors considered are age, gender, birth order and age of the mother. To test for any non-linearity, the square of the age of the child (Maxwell *et al.*, 2000) and of the mother have been introduced as explanatory variables. Further, an interactive dummy between gender and birth order has been constructed to see if there are gender effects which have been discussed in the literature by Behrman (1988a), Haddad (1987), Horton (1986), etc.

It is usually hypothesised that high birth order is associated with poor nutritional status of the young children as it increases the competition for the resources and maternal care within the family, as also concluded by Maxwell *et al.* (2000).

Age of the mother has been treated as a proxy for care taking abilities of the other. It is contended that too young mothers may not have enough experience to carry out the child rearing (Mishra *et al.*, 1999). Therefore, children born to younger mothers have higher risk of being malnourished.

Parent-specific Factors ($X_{h\ (p)}$)

The level of parental education, occupational status of the parents, power of the mother, nutritional status of the mother, and whether parents are living together or not are variables representing parent-specific caring behaviour for the children.

Education of mother is defined by three dummy variables representing less than middle level education, middle level education and equal to or more than high school level education—the reference category is mother with no education. Education of the mother is associated with better care giving resources and improving childcare practices as evident in studies of Horton (1988), Behrman and Deolalikar (1988), Haddad (1987) and McGuire and Popkin (1989). Some of the studies find strong negative impact of maternal education on breastfeeding, especially exclusive breastfeeding because of higher value of time (Guilkey and Stewart, 1995; Cebu study team, 1991; Wolfe and Behrman, 1987).

However, Sahn (1990) argues that a little variation in education levels or attending few years of school in the distant past may not make much difference to current functional abilities and thus, may not help in improving the nutritional status of the children significantly.

The level of father's education has been used as a variable to understand its effect on nutritional status of the preschool children, directly through income and indirectly through consumption preferences. Sahn (1990) and Alderman (1990) found that male preferences tended toward goods and services like entertainment, clothing, etc., which were less beneficial for children's nutrition in contrast to women's choices. This bias in preferences had a negative effect of father's education on nutritional status of children.

Occupational status of mother and father is another factor that affects the nutritional status of the children through caring practices. The nature of the mother's work affects the caring time and resources available to her. In this work, we introduce six dummy variables for working status of mother —highly skilled jobs, sales activities, agricultural labourer, self-employed in agriculture, manual skilled activities and manual unskilled activities as labourers, and the reference category is non-working women. Similarly, the occupational status of the father is represented through six dummy variables indicating that father involved in no work, highly skilled jobs, clerical work, sales activities, manual skilled activities and manual unskilled activities. The reference occupational group is self-employed in agriculture.

As discussed in section 2.3.3, the nutritional status of the mother has a bearing on the nutritional status of her preschool children (Martorell *et al.*, 1998; and WHO, 1995). This has been captured through a dummy variable which has a value 1 if BMI of the mother is less than 18.5 and 0 otherwise.

Woman's autonomy is represented through a dummy variable which takes a value 1 if mother takes decisions involving her health care on her own or jointly with her husband and 0 otherwise. It is argued in Smith *et al.* (2003) and Thomas (1997) that women with low status tend to have weaker control over household resources, tighter time constraints, less access to information and health services, poorer mental health, and lower self-esteem which affect the kind of care which they get and give to their children and thereby determine the nutritional status of children.

Whether husband and wife living together makes any difference to the nutritional status of the children has been captured through a dummy variable which takes a value 1 if couple lives together. Olaniyan (2002) suggests that living together means better social integration and better access to community resources and thus, translates into better nutritional status for children.

Household-specific Factors ($X_{h(r)}$)

Household factors considered in the model are demographic status (household size and composition) and socioeconomic status (size of the land holding, type of house, provision of electricity, sex of the head, religion and ethnicity) of the household. It also includes environmental factors related to source of water (pipe, pump, well and other sources) and provision of sanitation facilities.

Socioeconomic Status

It has been asserted in many studies as reviewed in Chapter 2 that key factor affecting all underlying determinants of malnutrition is low income or poverty (UNICEF, 1990). Therefore, one expects that nutritional status of an individual would be positively associated with per capita expenditure. Since NFHS does not provide information with regard to income of the household, we try to capture it through economic variables like size of the land holding, type of house, provision of electricity in the house, etc. Dummy variables are constructed to represent type of house—*pucca* and semi-*pucca*, while *kutcha* house is reference category. Similarly, supply of electricity is denoted by dummy variable having a value 1 if it has supply of electricity and 0 otherwise.

Ethnicity is represented by a dummy variable which takes a value 1 if household belongs to SC/ST/OBC category and 0 otherwise. Religion is represented by three dummy variables relating to religion of head of the households as Muslim, Christian and any other religion, while Hindu households are the reference households.

In keeping with the literature, the role of the head of the family has been analysed through a dummy variable which takes a value 1 if head is male and 0 otherwise.

Living Environment

The effect of unhygienic environment (water and sanitation) on morbidity and mortality through infections is well established in the literature (Checkley *et al.*, 2004; Esrey, 1996; Esrey *et al.*, 1992). Poor sanitation and water facility, and poor personal and environmental hygienic conditions are an important cause of infection—implying greater risk of illness and thus, malnourishment.

In this model, to see the effect of source of water, we have constructed three dummy variables for households using pipe, pump and well water. Households using any other source like spring, river, pond, and rainwater as source of water supply serve as reference category. Jalan and Ravallion (2001) found the positive health gains for children under the age of five years from piped water in rural India.

Whether purifying water has any effect on the nutritional status is captured by dummy variable which takes a value 1 if household is purifying water by using any means and 0 otherwise.

Provision of sanitary facilities is denoted by three dummy variables depending on whether household has its own toilet, shares a toilet, uses public toilet, where households having no toilet are the reference households. Esrey *et al.* (1992), McJunkin (1982) Anderson (1981) and Henry (1981) have shown the beneficial effect of sanitary conditions on the health of the individuals.

Demographic Variables

Size and composition of the household affect the level of care received by the children and thus, determine the nutritional status of the children. To analyse the effect of the household composition, household is decomposed into three groups *viz.* percentage of children in 0 to 5 years and 6 to 14 years and percentage of adult females, and the reference group is percentage of adult males. There is mixed evidence as far as issue of household size is concerned with positive coefficient (Sahn, 1990; Behrman and Wolfe, 1984) and negative coefficient (Melville *et al.*, 1988). It is generally believed that older siblings (six years and above) do not directly compete for nurturing time with younger child and provide some child care assistance which results in better nutritional status of the young child. Maxwell *et al.* (2000), Sahn (1990) etc., have found demographic age and sex groups to be significant.

Village–specific Factors (X_v)

The village-specific characteristics included in the model are accessibility to health facilities and sewerage system of the village. Access to health care infrastructure has been represented through dummy variable which takes a value 1 if health facility exists within village and 0 otherwise. Recent studies by Thomas *et al.* (1996) and Lavy *et al.* (1996) show that increasing provision of basic health services, that is, birth services, availability of drugs, immunisation, etc. improves the nutritional status of the children considerably.

Drainage facility in the village is represented by two dummy variables for open drainage and underground drainage, with no drainage system as the reference category. Various studies as reviewed in Chapter 2 have underlined the importance of sanitary conditions in influencing the health outcome of the individuals.

Thus, the variables used in explaining the weight-for-age z-score are summarised in Table 4.3.

Table 4.3

Correlates of Nutritional Status: Definitions of Explanatory Variables Used

Variable	*Definition*
Child-specific variables	
STBFEED	1 if the child is still being breastfed, and 0 otherwise.
OTHMILKDY	1 if other milk is taken daily, and 0 otherwise.
OTHMILKST	1 if other milk is taken sometimes, and 0 otherwise.
Reference category	1 if other milk is taken never, and 0 otherwise.
GLFDY	1 if green leafy vegetables are taken daily, and 0 otherwise.
GLFST	1 if green leafy vegetables are taken sometimes, and 0 otherwise.
Reference category	1 if green leafy vegetables are taken never, and 0 otherwise
FRTDY	1 if fruits are taken daily, and 0 otherwise.
FRTST	1 if fruits are taken sometimes, and 0 otherwise.
Reference category	1 if fruits are taken never, and 0 otherwise.
BM	0 refers to single birth, 1 refers to 1st of multiple, 2 refers to 2nd of multiple, 3 refers to 3rd of multiple.
GENDER	1 if child is male, and 0 otherwise.
BORD	Numeral 1,2, 3... where 1 refers to the oldest child in the family.

contd...

...contd...

AGE	Age of child is in (completed) months.
AGESQ	Square of age of child is in (completed) months.
MAGE	Age of the mother at the time of birth is in years (completed).
MSQAGE	Square of age of the mother at the time of birth is in (completed) years.
FEVER	Value 1 if child had fever, and 0 otherwise
DIAHHROEA	Value 1 if child had diarrhoea, and 0 otherwise.
Parent-specific variables	
LTOGETHER	1 if living together, and 0 otherwise.
MPOWER	1 if mother takes decisions involving her health care on her own or jointly with her husband, and 0 otherwise.
BMILT18	1 if body mass index less than 18.5, and 0 otherwise.
MEDUC1	1 if the mother has less than middle level education, and 0 otherwise.
MEDUC2	1 if the mother has middle level education, and 0 otherwise.
MEDUC3	1 if the mother has up to or more than high school level education, and 0 otherwise.
Reference category	1 if mother has no education, and 0 otherwise.
MOCCU1	1 if mother is involved in highly skilled jobs, and 0 otherwise.
MOCCU2	1 if mother is involved in sale activities, and 0 otherwise.
MOCCU3	1 if mother is working as agricultural labourer, and 0 otherwise.
MOCCU4	1 if mother is working as self-employed in agriculture, and 0 otherwise.
MOCCU5	1 if mother is involved in manual skilled activities, and 0 otherwise.
MOCCU6	1 if mother is involved in manual unskilled activities, and 0 otherwise.
Reference occupational group	1 if mother is not working, and 0 otherwise.
FEDU	Father's education 0,1,2,3, the level of class studied up to.
FOCCU0	1 if father is not working, and 0 otherwise.
FOCCU1	1 if father is involved in highly skilled jobs, and 0 otherwise.
FOCCU2	1 if father is clerk, and 0 otherwise
FOCCU3	1 if father is involved in sales activities and 0 otherwise.
FOCCU4	1 if father is engaged in manual skilled activities, and 0 otherwise.
FOCCU5	1 if father is involved in manual unskilled activities, and 0 otherwise.
Reference occupational group	1 if father is self-employed in agriculture, and 0 otherwise.

contd...

...contd...

Household-specific variables	
SCST	1 if household belongs to SC/ST/OBC category, and 0 otherwise.
MUSLIM	1 if Muslim, and 0 otherwise.
CHRISTIAN	1 if Christian, and 0 otherwise.
OTHRELIGION	1 if Sikh, Jain, Buddhist, etc., and 0 otherwise.
Reference religion	1 if Hindu, and 0 otherwise.
SEXHEAD	1 if head is male, and 0 otherwise.
HHSIZE	Numeral values indicate the total members in the family.
CHILD05	Percentage of children present in 0 to 5 years.
CHILD614	Percentage of children present in 6 to 14 years.
ADFEMALES	Percentage of females of 15 years and above.
Reference group	Percentage of males of 15 years and above.
SIZELAND	Size of the landholding (in acres of land).
PUCCA	1 if house is *pucca*, and 0 otherwise.
SEMIPUCCA	1 if house is semi-*pucca*, and 0 otherwise.
Reference house	1 if house is *kutcha*, and 0 otherwise.
ELECTRICITY	1 if it has supply of electricity, and 0 otherwise.
PIPE	1 if household has piped water, and 0 otherwise.
PUMP	1 if household has pumped water, and 0 otherwise.
WELL	1 if household has well water, and 0 otherwise.
Reference water source	1 if household has spring, river, pond, rainwater as source of water supply, and 0 otherwise.
PURIFY	1 if household is purifying water by using any means, and 0 otherwise.
OWNTOILET	1 if household has its own toilet, and 0 otherwise.
SHARETOILET	1 if household shares a toilet with others, and 0 otherwise.
PUBLICTOILET	1 if household uses public toilet, and 0 otherwise.
Reference toilet facility	1 if household has no toilet facility, and 0 otherwise.
Village–specific variables	
OPENDRAIN	1 if village has open drainage, and 0 otherwise.
UNDERDRAIN	1 if village has underground drainage, and 0 otherwise.
Reference drain system	1 if village has no drainage, and 0 otherwise.
HFVILAGE	1 if health facility exists within village, and 0 otherwise.

(b) Estimation Method

We introduce fixed-effect specification at state, village, household and parent levels and control for unobserved heterogeneity, and estimate the impact of the explanatory variables at the child, parent, household and village levels. This is implemented as follows:

(1) In the first step, using the parent fixed-effect specification, we regress NS_{ihv} on child-specific characteristics namely the age, gender, birth order, mother's age, breastfeeding, complementary food and health. Using these estimates of individual (child)-specific variables, we compute the fitted value for nutritional status, $\hat{NS}_{i(\overline{hv})}$

(2) In the second step, we compute the first set of residual (NS_{hv}) by taking away the effect of child-specific characteristics on NS_{ihv}.

$$NS_{hv} = NS_{ihv} - \hat{NS}_{i(\overline{hv})}$$

where NS_{ihv} is the observed standardised weight-for-age and $\hat{NS}_{i(\overline{hv})}$ is fitted value of the standardised weight-for-age using estimated values for child specific variables.

(3) In the third step, using the household fixed effect specification, we regress first set of residual NS_{hv} on the parent-specific variables $X_{h(p)}$ —education of mother and father, occupation of mother and father, power of mother, nutritional status of the mother and parents living together. Using estimated coefficient of parent-specific variables, we compute the fitted value of standardised weight-for-age, $\hat{NS}_{h(p)(\overline{h(r)v})}$

(4) In the fourth step, we compute second set of residuals which take away the effect of parent-specific variables $X_{h(p)}$ and child-specific variables (X_i) from standardised weight-for-age.

$$NS_{h(r)v} = NS_{hv} - \hat{NS}_{h(p)(\overline{h(r)v})}$$

(5) In the fifth step, using village fixed effect specification, the second set of residuals, $NS_{h(r)v}$, are regressed on the household resources variables —household size and composition, size of the land holding, type of house, provision of electricity, sex of the head, religion and ethnicity of the household. Using estimated coefficient of household resource-specific variables, we compute the fitted value of standardised weight-for-age, $\hat{NS}_{h(r)(\overline{v})}$

(6) In the sixth step, we compute third set of residuals, NS_v, which takes away the effect of household-specific (parent and resources) variables, X_h, and the child-specific variables, X_i, from standardised weight-for-age.

$$NS_v = NS_{h(r)v} - \hat{NS}_{h(p)(\overline{h(r)v})}$$

(7) In the seventh step, using state fixed-effect specification, these third set of residuals are regressed on the village level variables to estimate the coefficients of accessibility to health services and type of sewerage system.

4.4.2 Canonical Correlates of Nutritional Status of Mothers and Children

In the previous discussion, given the limitation of the NFHS data set, we have represented the nutrient intakes by frequency of intake of green leafy vegetables, fruits, mushy food or other milk rather than actual intakes of food or nutrient in determining nutritional status of the children.

In this part of the exercise, we take the advantage of the NSS data which has been used to derive estimates of nutrient intake (macro and micro) at the household level as described in section 3.2. Exploiting the near-coincidence of the NSS survey in 1999-2000 and the NFHS survey in 1998-99, we have constructed a data set with the NSS region as the unit of observation which can now correlate nutrient intakes and non-nutrient variables to the nutritional status as discussed in the section on merged data. We club the nutritional status for mothers and children together; however, it may be noted once again that these are cross-sectional data, with region-specific aggregates of nutritional status.

The objective of this part of research is to simply identify associations between set of nutritional status indicators which is represented by more than one indicator on one hand and nutrient intake and socioeconomic variables on the other hand by a multivariate statistical technique called canonical correlation. This technique helps us in identifying the components of one set of variables that are most highly related (linearly) to the components of the other set of variables.

While the familiar regression technique relates several independent variables to a single dependent variable, the canonical correlation can be used to analyse the relationship between two sets of variables. In this exercise, we have constructed two different sets of nutritional status of woman and children—in terms of prevalence of anthropometric failure and anaemia. We estimate the canonical correlations between the following:

NS_i (prevalence of anaemia among women, prevalence of anaemia among children)

= f_i (calories, iron, vitamin A, vitamin C, percentage of population having access to sanitation facilities, percentage of population using water purification methods, percentage of population having pump or pipe as source of drinking water, monthly per capita expenditure)

NS_i (percentage of women with BMI less than 18.5, percentage of children who are underweight)

= f_i (calories, iron, vitamin A, vitamin C, percentage of population having access to sanitation facilities, percentage of population using water purification methods, percentage of population having pump or pipe as source of drinking water, monthly per capita expenditure)

(a) Specification of Variables

Nutritional Status

In our study, we have used two important indicators of nutritional status of population: namely, prevalence of anthropometric failure and prevalence of anaemia among mothers and children from NFHS data.

Among children, as discussed in section 4.4.1, the anthropometric failure is captured by low weight-for-age variable, called underweight. The variable captures situations where a child does not eat an adequate amount of food relative to his needs, is ill, both of which result in a reduction of body weight. Children whose weight-for-age (z-score) is more than two standard deviations below the reference median weight-for-age are considered to be undernourished. Among adults, we have considered an individual as chronic energy deficient (CED) when she has BMI less than 18.5.[5]

Another popular indicator of nutritional status measured in terms of nutritional deficiency—anaemia is also available from NFHS data set. Since anaemia is a serious problem in case of women and children in terms of prevalence rate as well as severity, we chose it to represent a second set of nutritional status indicators. Thus, percentage of children under the age of three years who are anaemic and percentage of women who are anaemic form the second set of nutritional status indicators.

5. Since adults cannot grow, appropriate weight for actual height can be calculated to represent nutritional status adequately.

Nutrient Intakes

The average per capita per day intake of energy, iron, vitamin A and vitamin C are the nutrient intakes considered in the model. These variables are sourced from the NSS. Traditional models involving controlled study have focused on the positive effect of the per capita calorie (or protein) intakes on health outcomes (Chernichovsky and Kielmann, 1977 and Clark, 1981). 'It is an exception rather than rule to have a single nutritional deficiency' has been argued by Tomkins and Watson (1989: 13). It has also been highlighted in the recent literature where the importance of multi-micronutrient approach, especially emphasising the role of vitamin A and C, iron and zinc simultaneously than individually in improving growth of population, has been laid (Ramakrishnan *et al.*, 2004; Demment *et al.*, 2003; Rivera *et al.*, 2003; Gross *et al.*, 2000; Schultink and Gross, 1996).

The role of increased iron intakes and vitamin C in ameliorating nutritional anaemia has been documented (see for example, Bhargava, 2001). The importance of vitamin A has also been highlighted in reducing anaemia by Mwanri *et al.* (2000) and Schultink and Gross (1996).

In general, deficiency of these micronutrients causes growth faltering and reduces the immunity of the body, thus being more prone to bacterial and viral infections and diseases which adversely affect the nutritional status.

Living Environment

The state of sanitation and hygienic environments is captured by percentage of population having access to sanitation facilities. The variables constructed here are percentage of population using water purification methods and percentage of population having pump or pipe as source of drinking water (as an indicator of the availability of safe drinking water).

We expect that greater is the percentage of population having access to sanitation facilities and safe drinking water, the lower the prevalence of anaemia and undernourishment among the mothers and children. Scrimshaw *et al.* (1959) and others (for example, Bhargava, 2001) demonstrate that infectious diseases which are result of poor sanitary and unhygienic conditions often deplete the body's stores of vital nutrients such as iron. Further, the role of environmental factors has been emphasised as common cause of anaemia among the preschool children in studies of Asobayire *et al.* (2001), Brooker *et al.* (1999) and Stoltzfus *et al.* (1997). These variables have been constructed from the NFHS.

Income

As before, monthly per capita expenditure is used as an indicator of level of living of the household and is taken from the NSS; poverty remains the key factor behind the underlying determinants of nutritional status as indicated in Figure 1.1 (Chapter 1). Various studies have shown that low income or low standard of living is one of the important determinants of adverse nutritional outcomes (Strauss and Thomas (1998); Ricci and Becker (1996); Miller and Korenman (1994).

Thus, Tablc 4.4 providcs a key to the variables used in the canonical correlation analysis.

Table 4.4

Definitions of Variables Used in Canonical Correlation Analysis

Variable	*Definition*
Nutritional status indicators	
Variant 1	
Underweight among children (Y1)	% of children who have weight-for-age less than 2 SD
Underweight among women (Y2)	% of women who have BMI less than 18.5
Variant 2	
Anaemia among children (Y3)	% of children who have anaemia of any kind
Anaemia among women (Y4)	% of women who have anaemia of any kind
Nutrient intake	
Calories (X1)	Per capita per day intake of calories (kcal)
Iron (X2)	Per capita per day intake of iron (mg)
Vitamin A (X3)	Per capita per day intake of vitamin A (μg)
Vitamin C (X4)	Per capita per day intake of vitamin C (mg)
Socioeconomic status variables	
Incomc (X5)	Monthly per capita expenditure
Sanitation (X6)	% of population having access to sanitation facilities
Pump/Pipe (X7)	% of population having pump or pipe as source of drinking water
Purify water (X8)	% of population using water purification methods

(b) Estimation Method

Canonical correlation analysis explores the correlative structure of two sets of variables. Let us assume that variables in the first set be denoted as Y_1, Y_2 (the two nutritional status variables) and those in the second set be denoted, X_1, X_2, ...X_8 (nutrient and socioeconomic variables) .

The number of canonical correlations produced will be equal to two, the number of variables in the smaller data set of the two. The first pair of linear combination of two sets of variables is formed so that the correlation (R_{c1}) is maximised. Then, the second pair of linear combination is produced so that canonical correlation is also as large as possible but subject to the constraint that the second correlation (R_{c2}) is uncorrelated with the first correlation (R_{c1}). Subsequently, second correlation is always smaller than the first one.

In this exercise, canonical correlation defines Y canonical variate, a linear combination of *Y* variables,

$$Y = \alpha_1 Y_1 + \alpha_2 Y_2,$$

where Y_1 and Y_2 are prevalence of underweight among children and women respectively, and X canonical variate, linear combination of X variables,

$$X = \beta_1 X_1 + \beta_2 X_2 + ...\beta_8 X_8 ,$$

where X_1, X_2, X_3, X_4, are per capita intake of calories, iron, vitamin A and vitamin C respectively; X_5 is per capita income and X_6, X_7 and X_8 are percentage of population having sanitation facilities, pump/pipe as source of water, using purified water respectively. Here, α, is a set of weights chosen for Y set and β, is a set of weights chosen for X set which maximises the correlation between the two canonical variates, assuming X and Y are standardised.

The set of weights (β or α) produced above is called as loadings which is simple correlation between the original (X or Y) variate and its canonical variate. Although there are no rules for selecting which loadings are important for interpretation, it may be reasonable to consider loading below 0.40 as trivial, between 0.41 to 0.70 as moderate and above 0.70 as heavy (Laessig and Duckett, 1979).[6] Therefore, magnitude and sign of these loadings indicate the direction of the relationship between nutritional status and intakes.

Not all the correlation produced from the data set may be statistically significant. Just like any other correlation measure, R_{ci} is squared to give estimated total variance that is explained by the canonical variates chosen at that step. Its significance can be tested with the help of F-approximation devised by Rao or Chi-square approximation suggested by Bartlett.

Further, canonical correlation analysis gives the variance overlap or redundancy between the two sets of variables. Redundancy is obtained by the product of proportion of variance accounted for by canonical variate and proportion of total variance shared by the pair of canonical variates. It explains how much of the variance of Y (nutritional status) is obtainable from the knowledge of dietary-socioeconomic status variables. It is this feature of canonical correlation that we exploit the most in this analysis. (For details, refer to Bernstein *et al.*, 1988).

Similarly, second canonical correlation analysis is carried for both of the specifications outlined in section 4.4.2. The canonical correlation analysis is done using CANON and CANCOR command in STATA.

6. Laessig and Duckett (1979) have used this technique to identify association among health and environmental variables in Philadelphia.

5 Summarising Nutrient Intakes and Nutritional Status

In this part of the research work, we attempt to quantify the extent of deprivation in terms of nutrient intakes using the rich unit record data from the National Sample Survey Organisation's (NSSO) consumer expenditure surveys of 1983 and 1999-2000 for rural India. We also summarise data on the nutritional status of women between 15 and 49 years and children under the age of 3 years in 1998-99 in terms of anthropometric status and anaemia using the National Family Health Survey (NFHS) for rural India.

Of the various nutrients that are supplied through the food we eat, we extend the focus of nutrient deprivation from a focus on calorie, protein and fat (Meenakshi and Vishwanathan, 2001; Shariff and Mallick, 1999) to include micronutrients such as thiamine, riboflavin, niacin, vitamin A, vitamin C and iron. We present information disaggregated by state and quartile expenditure groups.

In this chapter, we: (i) track changes in dietary patterns, particularly with reference to dietary diversity, (ii) provide estimates of the quantum of intake of, as well as deprivation in, macro and micro nutrients for rural India and 15 major states individually at mean per capita income as well as at quartile incomes, (iii) examine how the magnitude of deprivation has changed between 1983 and 1999-2000, and (iv) summarise the evidence on nutritional status for adult women and children under three years of age in terms of anthropometric failure and anaemia in 1998-99.

5.1 Changes in Dietary Patterns

The period 1983 to 1999-2000 has seen substantial changes in food intake patterns in rural India. In particular, the share of cereals in total food expenditure has declined, while that of milk, meat, vegetables and fruits has increased (Figure 5.1). While these changes conform to Bennet's law, it is significant that these substitutions have occurred both among the rich and the poor. Thus, while, as expected, the top 25 per cent spends relatively greater amounts on milk, meat and so on, the decline in the share of staples is apparent among the poorest 25 per cent as well.

Figure 5.1

Share of Commodity Groups in Food Expenditure, by Quartile Expenditure Group, 1983 and 1999-2000

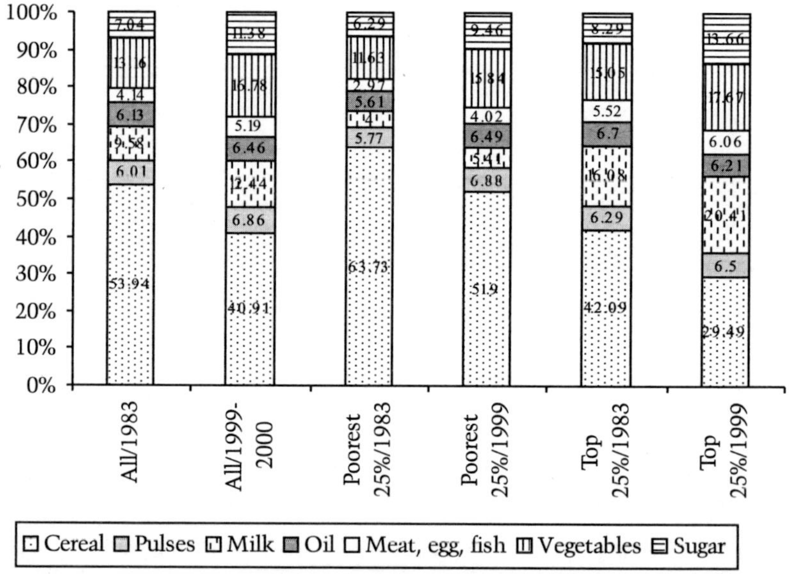

Source: Calculated from unit record data of the 38th and 55th NSSO rounds

This declining cereal share reflects a decreased intake of cereals in quantitative terms: cereal consumption declined from 14.8 kg in 1983 to 12.8 kg per capita per month between 1983 and 1999-2000. As indicated in Table 5.1, this fall is witnessed for both the poorest and the richest 25 per cent. Average per capita cereal intakes declined by over 4 kg per month for the top 25 per cent, and by 300 g for the poorest 25 per cent.

The state-level figures suggest that these decreases are fairly widespread: the agriculturally prosperous states of Punjab and Haryana saw average cereal intakes decline by 2.5–3 kg per capita per month, while declines of smaller magnitudes of 500 g may be seen in Kerala, Orissa and West Bengal.

Further, it is only in these three states and Bihar that an increase in cereal consumption among the poorest 25 per cent may be seen. It is no coincidence that apart from Kerala, these states rank among the poorest in the country.

Table 5.1

Per Capita Per Month Consumption of Cereals (Kilograms) across States and Quartiles

State	*All (1983)*	*All (1999-2000)*	*Poorest 25% (1983)*	*Poorest 25% 1999-2000)*	*Top 25% (1983)*	*Top 25% (1999-2000)*
Andhra Pradesh	15.4	12.8	12.5	10.7	18.4	14.6
Bihar	15.8	13.8	11.5	11.6	20.3	15.9
Gujarat	12.6	10.2	10.4	9.2	15.0	11.4
Haryana	14.6	11.4	11.7	10.0	18.6	12.6
Himachal Pradesh	16.1	12.9	13.1	11.8	18.7	13.8
Karnataka	15.1	11.6	10.9	9.4	19.3	13.9
Kerala	10.1	9.9	7.5	8.3	13.3	11.3
Madhya Pradesh	15.9	13.0	12.7	11.0	19.1	14.7
Maharashtra	13.8	11.4	11.9	10.1	15.9	12.2
Orissa	15.6	15.1	11.0	12.5	20.3	17.2
Punjab	13.6	10.6	10.3	9.2	17.6	12.5
Rajasthan	17.2	14.2	14.3	12.5	20.6	16.2
Tamil Nadu	13.1	10.7	9.4	8.8	17.0	12.5
Uttar Pradesh	15.5	13.6	12.1	12.0	18.9	15.3
West Bengal	14.3	13.6	9.5	10.9	19.0	15.8
Rural India	14.8	12.8	11.6	11.3	18.0	13.8

Source: Calculated from unit record data of the 38th and 55th NSSO rounds.

Accompanying the decreased dependence on cereals is an increase in dietary diversity. In our study, we define,

> Dietary diversity index (DDI) = Average number of commodities consumed as percentage of number of food items canvassed in the last 30 days in a particular household survey.

This normalisation has been done to ensure comparability, as the total number of food items canvassed between the two rounds has decreased. As evident in Table 5.2, the number of commodities consumed by the average rural household has nearly doubled between 1983 and 1999-2000 since the value of the index increased from 13.8 to 26.5.[1]

1. The corresponding unadjusted figures are: an average of 22.4 foods in 1983 (with 162 food items canvassed) and an average of 36.6 foods in 1999-2000 (with 138 food items canvassed).

This improvement in dietary diversity is substantiated by the percentage of sample households reporting positive consumption of milk and various fruits and vegetables. The 15-year period saw the percentage of sample households consuming fluid milk increase from 57 per cent to 68 per cent, those consuming fruits go up from 46 per cent to 68 per cent and a doubling of the percentage of sample households consuming tomatoes.

Table 5.2

Indicators of Diversifying Diets, Rural India, 1983 and 1999-2000

Variable	*1983*	*1999-2000*
A. Dietary Diversity Index	13.8	26.5
B. Percentage of sample households reporting consumption of		
Fluid milk	57	68
Fresh fruits	46	68
Onion	78	94
Tomatoes	30	64
Potatoes	80	93
C. Average intakes among consuming households: per capita per day consumption of		
Fluid milk (ml)	110	170
Green leafy vegetables (g)	30	25

Source: Calculated from unit record data of the 38th and 55th NSSO rounds

Despite this unambiguous evidence of diversification, it is important to note that a fairly high percentage of sample households—about one-third—report no consumption of fluid milk or of fruits in the previous 30 days. And while there is an improvement in the amount of intakes of fluid milk, even with the improvement, intakes are low compared with the 150 ml per day recommended for adults and the 250 ml per day recommended for children (Gopalan *et al.*, 2000).

Also noteworthy is the decline in the consumption of green leafy vegetables[2], an exception to the trend of increased consumption of fruits and vegetables. Further, diets continue to be cereal-based, with cereals accounting for 70 per cent of total energy intakes.

2. There is possibility that changes in the definition of green leafy vegetables are responsible for this decline. However, studies also suggest that exports of these vegetables have increased, perhaps at the expense of home consumption. See Vandana and Singh (2002).

The significance of improved dietary diversity for micronutrient intakes needs scarcely to be underlined. However, because diets are predominantly cereal-based and because the improvement in diversity is not of a sufficiently high order of magnitude, as we demonstrate later, these improvements are not reflected in improved micronutrient intakes (with few exceptions).

Indeed, to the extent that cereals are the principal source of several micronutrients including iron, niacin, thiamine and riboflavin, a decrease in cereal intakes has resulted into lower intakes of these micronutrients, despite the improvement in dietary diversity. This is documented in section 5.2.

5.2 Trends in Macronutrients and Micronutrients

Given this background on changes in dietary patterns, we turn now to examination of trends in incidence, depth and severity of undernutrition with respect to both macronutrients and micronutrients. But first we examine major sources of these nutrients (Table 5.3) as this information, along with changes in the dietary patterns just outlined, helps in interpreting the observed trends. A disaggregation by quartile expenditure group and by year is presented in Appendix Table A-5.1.1.

Table 5.3

Contribution of Various Foods to Nutrient Intakes (%), 1999-2000

Food Group	*Calories*	*Protein*	*Fat*	*Iron*	*Vitamin C*	*Vitamin A*	*Thiamine*	*Niacin*	*Riboflavin*
Cereals	69.1	68.7	17.4	76.4	0.4	9.9	77.0	85.1	64.4
Pulses	4.4	10.6	1.6	5.2	0.2	4.1	7.0	4.0	4.9
Milk and milk products	5.8	7.8	20.9	1.2	4.3	19.2	3.1	0.7	14.6
Meat, egg and fish	0.8	4.0	2.0	1.1	0.3	3.1	0.9	0.7	1.8
Vegetables and fruits	6.1	6.4	5.4	8.9	91.0	55.0	9.6	6.4	11.8
Oils	6.6	0.0	49.0	0.0	0.0	2.4	0.1	0.1	0.0
Other food	7.2	2.5	3.6	7.3	3.9	5.5	2.3	2.3	2.5

Source: Calculated from unit record data of the 55th NSSO round.

The evidence in Table 5.3 indicates the overwhelming dependence of rural diets on cereals as the principal source of many nutrients. Thus, nearly two-thirds of energy, protein and riboflavin are accounted for by cereals, and over three-fourths of the intakes of niacin, thiamine and iron are from the consumption of cereals. Cereals also account for a significant share of fat intakes. The only exceptions are vitamin A and vitamin C, the principal sources of which are fresh fruits and vegetables.

With a shift in diets from cereals to non-cereal foods, the share of cereals in calories, proteins, thiamine, riboflavin and niacin has reduced, while that of non-cereal food items like milk and its products, vegetables, fruits, oils, etc., has increased. This has occurred not only among the richest but also among the poorest quartile as observed in Appendix Table A-5.1.1. However, the magnitude of change is much larger for the rich than poor.

5.2.1 Energy

Table 5.4 sets out trends in average intakes and head count ratios (HCR) of inadequate energy intakes. Average intakes decreased from 2260 kcal/day to 2145 kcal/day[3], translating into an increase in HCR from 41 per cent to 48 per cent between 1983 and 1999-2000.

The decreased consumption of cereals and the reliance on cereals as the principal source of energy account for this decline; the increases in non-cereal foods have not been of a sufficiently high order of magnitude to affect this decline. This implies that even after several decades of being self-sufficient in food grains, nearly half of India's rural population has energy intakes that are less than the recommended dietary allowance (RDA).

In general, states of Haryana, Himachal Pradesh, Rajasthan, Punjab and Uttar Pradesh enjoy better energy intakes and thus, lower levels of deficiency than in other states where more than half of the population is calorie deficient. At the same time, as indicated in Table 5.5, the Foster-Greek-Thorbecke (FGT) (1) and FGT (2) measures are indicative of an improvement in the average gap and severity of energy inadequacy in most of the states except Andhra Pradesh, Maharashtra and Madhya Pradesh.

---

3. It is important to note that these are slightly different from those in the published reports of the NSS on account of commodity coverage as discussed in section 3.2.

Table 5.4

Average Calorie Intakes and Incidence of Calorie Deprivation, by Quartile Expenditure Group, between 1983 and 1999-2000

State	Calorie Intakes (kcal per capita per day)						Incidence of Calorie Deprivation (%) (HCR)					
	1983			1999-2000			1983			1999-2000		
	Poorest 25%	Top 25%	All	Poorest 25%	Top 25%	All	Poorest 25%	Top 25%	All	Poorest 25%	Top 25%	All
Andhra Pradesh	1663	3062	2302	1575	2541	2029	73.8	9.7	37.1	90.0	20.7	56.0
Bihar	1501	3023	2211	1641	2668	2116	87.1	4.8	40.3	83.8	12.7	47.0
Gujarat	1604	2893	2176	1572	2530	2004	80.8	13.1	45.8	88.1	20.9	56.5
Haryana	1818	3730	2612	1792	3190	2460	60.2	1.6	25.1	75.8	4.2	31.5
Himachal Pradesh	1982	3529	2710	1995	3009	2460	44.9	5.7	18.3	61.6	7.2	25.8
Karnataka	1485	3117	2260	1492	2614	2029	84.3	13.0	43.8	91.0	23.7	58.0
Kerala	1222	2715	1868	1449	2599	2006	98.7	18.8	66.7	96.6	19.1	58.9
Madhya Pradesh	1690	3177	2342	1568	2641	2059	72.9	6.5	33.7	88.7	18.2	53.1
Maharashtra	1681	2765	2160	1606	2459	2020	75.8	17.9	45.9	87.0	27.7	56.9
Orissa	1383	2919	2109	1641	2662	2142	94.2	5.2	48.3	83.2	11.6	45.1
Punjab	1814	3788	2699	1789	3187	2393	62.8	4.4	25.3	71.8	3.7	32.9
Rajasthan	1862	3615	2609	1882	3086	2423	55.6	4.6	24.4	56.5	5.3	24.9
Tamil Nadu	1222	2775	1920	1346	2383	1836	96.7	23.0	64.0	97.2	37.2	71.4
Uttar Pradesh	1718	3396	2466	1804	2997	2331	69.7	5.7	30.5	66.8	8.0	33.8
West Bengal	1254	2946	2042	1611	2650	2107	74.8	10.1	55.4	85.4	15.9	49.6
Rural India	1580	3083	2262	1660	2690	2145	78.8	11.2	41.5	80.2	19.3	48.0

Source: Calculated from unit record data of the 38th and 55th NSSO rounds

When trends disaggregated by income groups are examined, among the poorest 25 per cent, average intakes increased in Bihar, Kerala, Orissa and Uttar Pradesh. These states thus saw a decrease in the incidence of calorie deprivation given by HCR among the poor. Three of these states rank among the poorest in the country. It is no coincidence that these states also saw an increased consumption of cereals between 1983 and 1999-2000. Thus, the poorest 25 per cent in the poorest states saw improved energy intakes.

On the other hand, caloric intakes among the poorest 25 per cent declined in Andhra Pradesh, Gujarat, Haryana, Punjab, Maharashtra and Madhya Pradesh; many of these states are relatively more prosperous.

Table 5.5

Depth and Severity of Calorie Deprivation, by Quartile Expenditure Group, between 1983 and 1999-2000

State	Depth of Calorie Deprivation (FGT [1])						Severity of Calorie Deprivation Gap (FGT [2])					
	1983			1999-2000			1983			1999-2000		
	Poorest 25%	Top 25%	All	Poorest 25%	Top 25%	All	Poorest 25%	Top 25%	All	Poorest 25%	Top 25%	All
Andhra Pradesh	0.18	0.01	0.07	0.22	0.02	0.10	0.06	0.00	0.02	0.07	0.00	0.03
Bihar	0.23	0.00	0.08	0.18	0.01	0.08	0.08	0.00	0.03	0.05	0.00	0.02
Gujarat	0.20	0.02	0.09	0.21	0.03	0.11	0.07	0.01	0.03	0.07	0.00	0.03
Haryana	0.13	0.00	0.05	0.13	0.00	0.05	0.05	0.00	0.02	0.03	0.00	0.01
Himachal Pradesh	0.10	0.01	0.04	0.07	0.01	0.03	0.04	0.00	0.01	0.01	0.00	0.01
Karnataka	0.25	0.02	0.10	0.25	0.03	0.12	0.10	0.01	0.04	0.09	0.01	0.04
Kerala	0.38	0.03	0.18	0.28	0.02	0.12	0.16	0.01	0.07	0.10	0.00	0.04
Madhya Pradesh	0.16	0.01	0.06	0.22	0.02	0.10	0.05	0.00	0.02	0.07	0.00	0.03
Maharashtra	0.17	0.03	0.08	0.22	0.04	0.10	0.05	0.01	0.02	0.07	0.01	0.03
Orissa	0.30	0.01	0.11	0.17	0.01	0.07	0.12	0.00	0.04	0.05	0.00	0.02
Punjab	0.14	0.01	0.05	0.13	0.00	0.05	0.05	0.00	0.02	0.03	0.00	0.01
Rajasthan	0.11	0.01	0.04	0.09	0.01	0.03	0.04	0.00	0.02	0.02	0.00	0.01
Tamil Nadu	0.38	0.03	0.17	0.32	0.05	0.17	0.18	0.01	0.07	0.12	0.01	0.06
Uttar Pradesh	0.15	0.01	0.06	0.13	0.01	0.05	0.05	0.00	0.02	0.04	0.00	0.01
West Bengal	0.36	0.02	0.14	0.20	0.02	0.09	0.17	0.01	0.06	0.06	0.00	0.02
Rural India	0.21	0.02	0.09	0.18	0.03	0.09	0.08	0.00	0.03	0.06	0.01	0.02

Source: Calculated from unit record data of the 38th and 55th NSSO rounds

The picture with respect to the average calorie gap and severity of calorie deficiency is also mixed for the poorest 25 per cent. Andhra Pradesh, Gujarat, Haryana, Punjab, Maharashtra and Madhya Pradesh showed the rise in the extent of the calorie gap, while severity of the gap has increased only in Andhra Pradesh, Madhya Pradesh and Maharashtra.

Among the richest 25 per cent, average intakes have declined unambiguously, leading to an increase in the HCR and gap over time. In absolute terms, as expected, the HCR, FGT (1) and FGT (2) figures are all much lower for the richest 25 per cent than the poorest.

5.2.2 Protein

As was the case with the calories, the increased protein intakes from milk and its products, vegetables, meat, etc., have not been able to offset the substantial fall from cereal proteins, resulting in a decline of 4.9 g in per capita per day protein intake as seen in Appendix Table A-5.1.2. The average rural per capita per day protein intake decreased from 65 g in 1983 to 59.5 g in 1999-2000, increasing the HCR of protein deficiency from 30 per cent to 37.5 per cent, more than one-third of the population is protein deficient (Table 5.6).

Table 5.6

Average Protein Intakes and Incidence of Protein Deprivation, by Quartile Expenditure Group, between 1983 and 1999-2000

State	Protein Intakes (g per capita per day)						Incidence of Protein Deprivation (%) (HCR)					
	1983			1999/2000			1983			1999/2000		
	Poorest 25%	Top 25%	All	Poorest 25%	Top 25%	All	Poorest 25%	Top 25%	All	Poorest 25%	Top 25%	All
Andhra Pradesh	44.0	85.2	62.2	39.8	63.8	50.2	62.0	10.0	33.3	86.9	27.5	60.8
Bihar	46.5	88.4	66.1	45.1	75.0	58.8	50.7	2.6	21.3	58.4	7.3	31.2
Gujarat	47.6	83.1	63.4	45.8	68.9	55.7	52.7	11.3	28.5	65.7	19.1	42.9
Haryana	57.0	114.8	81.5	54.5	96.3	75.6	25.0	0.9	9.9	37.2	5.4	14.6
Himachal Pradesh	63.3	108.8	84.8	61.0	88.2	74.0	18.7	3.0	8.0	23.1	4.0	10.3
Karnataka	41.0	82.8	60.9	40.5	69.3	54.4	69.3	12.2	36.9	72.7	22.4	49.3
Kerala	30.3	73.0	48.4	36.0	72.2	53.2	96.4	20.0	64.5	94.4	14.0	54.5
Madhya Pradesh	51.1	94.2	69.3	43.5	75.4	58.4	42.3	3.2	19.9	68.7	12.1	37.3
Maharashtra	49.5	79.7	62.7	45.0	69.6	57.4	43.5	10.1	26.4	64.1	21.2	39.2
Orissa	33.1	73.5	51.9	37.6	66.0	50.8	94.3	7.0	50.9	88.1	19.3	57.4
Punjab	55.1	112.1	81.1	54.9	96.4	72.4	31.2	3.0	12.6	32.6	1.5	14.1
Rajasthan	61.2	113.2	83.5	61.2	99.6	78.7	18.4	2.7	8.1	14.5	1.9	5.7
Tamil Nadu	32.5	73.3	50.3	32.3	61.2	45.4	89.1	19.1	58.2	96.0	38.3	73.0
Uttar Pradesh	54.4	105.9	77.0	53.4	88.9	69.7	33.2	2.0	12.8	31.3	3.2	13.6
West Bengal	33.5	75.9	52.8	38.5	67.5	52.2	89.7	12.1	50.2	83.3	19.0	51.8
Rural India	45.2	88.2	64.5	45.0	76.1	59.6	54.5	9.0	29.6	62.2	16.0	37.6

Source: Calculated from unit record data of the 38th and 55th NSSO rounds.

Intake of animal proteins (from milk, meat, egg, and fish) has increased by 1 g over time (Appendix Table A-5.1.2). Animal proteins such as milk, egg, and fish are considered to be of higher quality than vegetable proteins, as noted in Chapter 3.

In general, states of Haryana, Himachal Pradesh, Punjab, Rajasthan, Uttar Pradesh and Bihar have higher protein intakes than states of Karnataka, Kerala, Andhra Pradesh, Tamil Nadu, West Bengal and Orissa. Thus, incidence of protein deficiency is of much lower magnitude in the northern states than in the other states.

In comparison to 1983, average protein intakes declined in all states except Kerala. This decrease in protein intakes has resulted in increase in incidence of protein deficiency among all states except Kerala and Rajasthan.

Focusing on the poorest 25 per cent indicates there has been a decrease in proportion of population not getting the required minimum protein intakes only in the poorer states of Kerala, Orissa, West Bengal, Rajasthan and Uttar Pradesh[4] which had experienced either increase or marginal fall in per capita cereal consumption. However, the top quartile has witnessed a decline in protein intakes in all states primarily on account of substantial fall in cereal intake. Still the prevalence of inadequate intakes is much higher among the poor (62%) as compared to the rich (16%).

While the measure of inadequacy FGT (1) shows no change, FGT (2) has declined from 0.024 to 0.021 for rural India as evident in Table 5.7. However, there are differences in the performance of states, as half of the states exhibit an increase in depth and severity of protein gap, while the other half witnessed a decline. The number of states exhibiting worsening of depth and severity of protein deprivation is fewer for the poorest quartile than for the richest quartile.

As discussed earlier, the consequences of declining protein intakes may be offset, at least in small measure, by improvements in the quality of protein intakes.

4. UP had very small fall of 100 gms in per capita per month cereals intake.

Table 5.7

Depth and Severity of Protein Deprivation, by Quartile Expenditure Group, between 1983 and 1999-2000

State	Depth of Protein Deprivation (FGT (1))						Severity of Protein Deprivation (FGT(2))					
	1983			1999-2000			1983			1999-2000		
	Poorest 25%	Top 25%	All	Poorest 25%	Top 25%	All	Poorest 25%	Top 25%	All	Poorest 25%	Top 25%	All
Andhra Pradesh	0.158	0.013	0.067	0.238	0.034	0.122	0.056	0.004	0.021	0.083	0.007	0.035
Bihar	0.119	0.003	0.042	0.119	0.008	0.05	0.042	0.001	0.013	0.035	0.001	0.013
Gujarat	0.124	0.019	0.055	0.147	0.026	0.077	0.045	0.006	0.018	0.045	0.005	0.021
Haryana	0.063	0.002	0.023	0.044	0.005	0.016	0.031	0.00	0.011	0.008	0.001	0.003
Himachal Pradesh	0.048	0.006	0.018	0.025	0.004	0.01	0.022	0.002	0.008	0.005	0.001	0.002
Karnataka	0.196	0.023	0.084	0.191	0.029	0.101	0.081	0.007	0.03	0.067	0.007	0.031
Kerala	0.378	0.033	0.185	0.29	0.021	0.129	0.171	0.009	0.071	0.111	0.006	0.043
Madhya Pradesh	0.095	0.005	0.037	0.158	0.016	0.072	0.034	0.001	0.012	0.051	0.004	0.021
Maharashtra	0.087	0.016	0.045	0.15	0.026	0.071	0.028	0.005	0.013	0.05	0.005	0.02
Orissa	0.312	0.008	0.118	0.214	0.021	0.105	0.131	0.002	0.042	0.067	0.004	0.028
Punjab	0.077	0.005	0.032	0.045	0.002	0.018	0.037	0.002	0.015	0.012	0.001	0.004
Rajasthan	0.039	0.009	0.017	0.019	0.002	0.007	0.019	0.004	0.008	0.005	0.000	0.002
Tamil Nadu	0.336	0.03	0.157	0.344	0.06	0.19	0.158	0.007	0.061	0.143	0.015	0.067
Uttar Pradesh	0.063	0.003	0.023	0.054	0.003	0.02	0.022	0.001	0.008	0.016	0.001	0.005
West Bengal	0.308	0.018	0.124	0.216	0.022	0.098	0.135	0.005	0.047	0.074	0.004	0.028
Rural India	0.151	0.015	0.07	0.148	0.023	0.07	0.062	0.004	0.024	0.05	0.006	0.021

Source: Calculated from unit record data of the 38th and 55th NSSO rounds

5.2.3 Fat

Unlike the other two macronutrients, fat intakes have increased from 28.8 gms to 35.7 gms per capita per day in rural India (Table 5.8). This increase can be observed in virtually all states. Fats derived from cereals and pulses are termed 'invisible fats', while those derived from vegetable oils and ghee are termed 'visible'. As shown in Table 5.3, the increase in average intakes is entirely on account of the visible fats, and has occurred despite a reduction in the share of invisible fats.

Along with the increase in fat intake, the depth and severity of the fat deprivation has reduced in all states and across all quartiles except Andhra Pradesh,[5] as is evident from Table 5.8 and Table 5.9. There are significant

5. The average fat intake for the upper half of the population has decreased marginally.

variations in fat intake among states. The average per capita *per diem* fat intake among richer states of Punjab and Haryana is as high as 60 g, while the same for Orissa is 16.6 gms and for Bihar is 25.8 g in 1999-2000.

Table 5.8

Average Fat Intakes and Incidence of Fat Deprivation, by Quartile Expenditure Group, between 1983 and 1999-2000

	Fat Intakes (g per capita per day)						*Incidence of Fat Deprivation (%) (HCR)*					
	1983			*1999-2000*			*1983*			*1999-2000*		
State	*Poorest 25%*	*Top 25%*	*All*	*Poorest 25%*	*Top 25%*	*All*	*Poorest 25%*	*Top 25%*	*All*	*Poorest 25%*	*Top 25%*	*All*
Andhra Pradesh	15.2	49.9	29.8	18.4	45.3	29.8	98.1	54.1	80.6	100.0	45.1	82.4
Bihar	12.9	32.7	20.6	15.3	40.7	25.8	99.3	77.9	93.4	100.0	62.9	89.3
Gujarat	29.0	72.5	48.0	34.1	77.8	54.2	87.8	9.0	45.5	76.1	2.3	29.5
Haryana	25.1	85.4	50.8	33.8	89.2	59.3	93.2	8.6	48.2	73.9	2.3	28.2
Himachal Pradesh	31.2	77.8	51.8	36.3	79.3	54.8	83.3	9.3	42.6	82.4	5.7	36.7
Karnataka	14.0	41.9	26.2	23.2	52.0	36.6	99.7	61.8	86.7	98.1	30.5	70.6
Kerala	11.8	45.8	25.4	23.5	60.6	39.3	99.7	48.9	85.3	98.0	13.9	61.2
Madhya Pradesh	14.4	47.0	26.3	18.6	51.4	31.2	100.0	50.9	84.7	99.3	39.4	78.6
Maharashtra	18.2	47.6	30.1	26.2	58.1	39.6	99.5	45.8	81.1	96.4	21.2	61.9
Orissa	5.7	23.2	12.8	9.3	27.0	16.6	100.0	90.5	97.6	99.8	87.4	96.4
Punjab	28.1	86.0	54.0	36.9	88.3	59.2	86.8	9.9	42.1	70.0	2.8	27.7
Rajasthan	25.3	81.0	48.6	33.0	79.4	53.6	91.7	14.4	51.1	79.1	4.1	35.2
Tamil Nadu	11.1	39.3	22.2	17.4	45.7	29.7	100.0	66.1	90.1	99.8	45.8	82.3
Uttar Pradesh	15.8	59.2	33.0	22.9	61.8	37.9	98.2	40.1	76.5	98.1	26.9	70.6
West Bengal	8.1	31.3	17.3	14.3	40.1	24.4	99.1	80.1	94.8	99.3	71.8	91.5
Rural India	14.5	50.5	28.8	19.3	57.8	35.7	99.2	49.1	80.8	98.3	29.9	71.5

Source: Calculated from unit record data of the 38th and 55th NSSO rounds

Also there is a wide range of intakes across quartiles—average intakes for the poorest 25 per cent were 19.3 g per day, while those for richest 25 per cent were as high as 57.8 g per day. Therefore, despite an increase of nearly 5 g in the average intakes of the poorest 25 per cent, there has been a less than 1 per cent decrease in HCR of inadequate fat intakes; virtually all people in the poorest expenditure quartile have insufficient fat intakes. Similarly, despite the substantial increase in intakes among the richest 25 per cent, HCR remain as high as 30 per cent even in 1999-2000. It is only in states of Gujarat, Haryana and Punjab that there is virtually no inadequacy among the richest 25 per cent. Indeed, in these states, the problem may even be one of over nutrition as average fat intakes among the rich are twice the RDA.

Table 5.9

Depth and Severity of Fat Deprivation, by Quartile Expenditure Group, between 1983 and 1999-2000

State	*Depth of Fat Deprivation (FGT (1))*						*Severity of Fat Deprivation (FGT(2))*					
	1983			*1999-2000*			*1983*			*1999-2000*		
	Poorest 25%	*Top 25%*	*All*	*Poorest 25%*	*Top 25%*	*All*	*Poorest 25%*	*Top 25%*	*All*	*Poorest 25%*	*Top 25%*	*All*
Andhra Pradesh	0.63	0.18	0.41	0.56	0.10	0.33	0.44	0.08	0.26	0.33	0.03	0.18
Bihar	0.68	0.28	0.48	0.64	0.17	0.40	0.48	0.13	0.31	0.42	0.06	0.24
Gujarat	0.33	0.02	0.17	0.21	0.00	0.11	0.16	0.01	0.08	0.08	0.00	0.04
Haryana	0.39	0.02	0.21	0.22	0.00	0.11	0.20	0.01	0.10	0.09	0.00	0.04
Himachal Pradesh	0.29	0.02	0.15	0.23	0.01	0.12	0.13	0.01	0.07	0.08	0.00	0.04
Karnataka	0.65	0.20	0.43	0.43	0.05	0.24	0.45	0.09	0.27	0.22	0.02	0.12
Kerala	0.71	0.13	0.42	0.42	0.02	0.22	0.52	0.05	0.29	0.21	0.01	0.11
Madhya Pradesh	0.65	0.17	0.41	0.59	0.10	0.35	0.45	0.08	0.27	0.39	0.04	0.21
Maharashtra	0.55	0.12	0.33	0.43	0.03	0.23	0.32	0.04	0.18	0.22	0.01	0.12
Orissa	0.86	0.46	0.66	0.77	0.37	0.57	0.74	0.27	0.51	0.61	0.18	0.40
Punjab	0.33	0.01	0.17	0.18	0.00	0.09	0.16	0.00	0.08	0.06	0.00	0.03
Rajasthan	0.40	0.03	0.22	0.23	0.01	0.12	0.22	0.01	0.11	0.09	0.00	0.05
Tamil Nadu	0.72	0.25	0.48	0.58	0.11	0.34	0.55	0.12	0.33	0.35	0.04	0.19
Uttar Pradesh	0.61	0.12	0.36	0.51	0.06	0.28	0.40	0.05	0.23	0.29	0.02	0.15
West Bengal	0.80	0.32	0.56	0.65	0.21	0.43	0.65	0.16	0.40	0.44	0.08	0.26
Rural India	0.65	0.17	0.41	0.56	0.07	0.31	0.46	0.08	0.27	0.35	0.03	0.19

Source: Calculated from unit record data of the 38th and 55th NSSO rounds

5.2.4 Iron

Average iron intakes declined by 3 mg per capita per day between 1983 and 1999-2000 as indicated in Table 5.10. This is almost entirely on account of declining cereal intakes which account for the bulk of dietary intakes of iron. While iron from meat, eggs and fish increased slightly over this period, these sources of iron continue to constitute a relatively small share of total iron intakes. Also the reliance on vegetables and fruits has increased slightly (Table 5.3).

Of significance is the lack of improvement in iron derived from green leafy vegetables. While there is some evidence to suggest that the consumption of green leafy vegetables has declined, a part of the explanation may also lie in the changed definitions of commodities between 1983 and 1999-2000 rounds. In the NSS household questionnaire canvassed in 1983, *palak* was listed separately from 'other leafy vegetables' in the list of vegetables consumed over the past 30 days. However, in 1999-2000, these two categories of vegetables were merged as 'other leafy vegetables'. It is possible that as a consequence, there may be under reporting of the total consumption of green leafy vegetables, although it is not possible to quantify this.

Table 5.10

Average Iron Intakes and Incidence of Iron Deprivation, by Quartile Expenditure Group, between 1983 and 1999-2000

	Iron Intakes (mg per capita per day)						*Incidence of Iron Deprivation (%) (HCR)*					
	1983			*1999-2000*			*1983*			*1999-2000*		
State	*Poorest 25%*	*Top 25%*	*All*	*Poorest 25%*	*Top 25%*	*All*	*Poorest 25%*	*Top 25%*	*All*	*Poorest 25%*	*Top 25%*	*All*
Andhra Pradesh	18.8	30.3	24.0	15.7	23.8	19.5	83.7	46.9	68.0	97.7	82.3	92.3
Bihar	19.0	34.5	26.2	18.9	30.9	24.7	83.8	24.6	55.6	89.8	38.1	65.4
Gujarat	21.5	36.2	28.8	18.9	28.2	23.4	69.1	31.1	47.6	85.0	58.6	71.5
Haryana	23.7	41.8	31.7	20.3	28.6	24.7	60.8	11.3	38.4	86.5	49.3	67.3
Himachal Pradesh	19.4	33.6	26.2	19.5	26.8	22.9	76.6	36.0	53.7	92.1	68.8	82.0
Karnataka	17.6	34.1	25.3	15.8	25.8	20.8	87.0	33.2	61.0	95.9	70.3	84.6
Kerala	12.0	26.7	18.5	14.2	25.5	20.0	99.6	63.6	89.1	99.4	72.2	89.3
Madhya Pradesh	19.7	35.2	26.4	17.2	28.5	22.6	79.8	26.1	55.1	94.7	53.8	74.8
Maharashtra	20.5	30.9	25.3	18.5	25.7	22.3	80.1	46.0	63.5	89.9	70.3	79.7
Orissa	16.9	33.5	24.6	17.4	30	23.5	93.7	25.8	64.9	96.0	47.8	77.5
Punjab	21.1	39.4	29.4	19.7	31.2	24.7	71.9	21.2	44.9	87.4	43.7	70.3
Rajasthan	18.3	46.1	33.2	23.5	35.3	29.4	72.3	13.6	38.5	62.4	26.8	43.8
Tamil Nadu	12.9	30.1	21.4	13.3	22.6	17.8	91.9	56.7	76.5	99.8	85.0	94.7
Uttar Pradesh	22	38.4	29.5	21.9	32.1	26.6	69.5	18.8	42.2	74.9	37.8	56.0
West Bengal	16.5	34.3	24.5	17.8	28.8	23.0	91.9	29.0	67.2	95.1	52.1	77.1
Rural India	19.1	34.3	26.2	18.7	28.2	23.0	80.2	34.0	57.8	88.4	57.4	73.0

Source: Calculated from unit record data of the 38th and 55th NSSO rounds

Thus, between 1983 and 1999-2000, average iron intakes declined in all states except Kerala. The magnitude of the decrease varies directly with the fall in cereal intakes. The richer states of Punjab and Haryana saw a decrease of nearly 5-7 mg per capita per day, whereas the poor states of Bihar and Orissa, where the decline in cereal intake was more modest, saw a decline of 1-1.5 mg per capita per day.

Correspondingly, the incidence of iron deficiency has increased. At the all India level, a 3 mg decrease in average intakes has resulted in an increase in HCR of nearly 15 percentage points. The increase is as high as 25-30 percentage points in states such as Haryana, Punjab and Gujarat.

Table 5.11

Depth and Severity of Iron Deprivation, by Quartile Expenditure Group, between 1983 and 1999-2000

State	*Depth of Iron Deprivation (FGT (1))*						*Severity of Iron Deprivation (FGT(2))*					
	1983			*1999-2000*			*1983*			*1999-2000*		
	Poorest 25%	*Top 25%*	*All*	*Poorest 25%*	*Top 25%*	*All*	*Poorest 25%*	*Top 25%*	*All*	*Poorest 25%*	*Top 25%*	*All*
Andhra Pradesh	0.28	0.09	0.17	0.41	0.2	0.3	0.12	0.03	0.06	0.19	0.07	0.12
Bihar	0.27	0.03	0.13	0.26	0.06	0.15	0.12	0.01	0.05	0.10	0.01	0.05
Gujarat	0.25	0.07	0.14	0.32	0.14	0.22	0.12	0.03	0.06	0.15	0.05	0.09
Haryana	0.16	0.03	0.09	0.24	0.1	0.16	0.08	0.01	0.04	0.08	0.03	0.05
Himachal Pradesh	0.28	0.07	0.15	0.26	0.13	0.19	0.15	0.02	0.06	0.10	0.04	0.06
Karnataka	0.31	0.07	0.17	0.38	0.17	0.27	0.15	0.02	0.07	0.18	0.06	0.11
Kerala	0.53	0.14	0.35	0.48	0.17	0.31	0.30	0.04	0.16	0.24	0.05	0.13
Madhya Pradesh	0.24	0.04	0.13	0.34	0.11	0.21	0.10	0.01	0.05	0.15	0.03	0.08
Maharashtra	0.23	0.09	0.16	0.3	0.17	0.22	0.09	0.03	0.05	0.13	0.05	0.08
Orissa	0.35	0.03	0.17	0.32	0.08	0.19	0.16	0.01	0.06	0.12	0.02	0.06
Punjab	0.22	0.05	0.12	0.25	0.08	0.16	0.11	0.02	0.05	0.09	0.02	0.05
Rajasthan	0.4	0.03	0.15	0.17	0.05	0.1	0.31	0.01	0.10	0.07	0.01	0.03
Tamil Nadu	0.51	0.13	0.28	0.49	0.25	0.37	0.35	0.04	0.15	0.26	0.09	0.17
Uttar Pradesh	0.19	0.03	0.09	0.18	0.06	0.11	0.07	0.01	0.03	0.06	0.01	0.03
West Bengal	0.37	0.05	0.18	0.33	0.1	0.2	0.18	0.01	0.07	0.14	0.03	0.07
Rural India	0.29	0.07	0.16	0.29	0.13	0.2	0.14	0.03	0.07	0.12	0.04	0.07

Source: Calculated from unit record data of the 38th and 55th NSSO rounds

Quartile-specific trends are similar. Iron intakes declined by as much as 6 mg per capita per day among the richest 25 per cent as compared to 0.4 mg for the poorest 25 per cent. This has meant a doubling of incidence of iron insufficiency among the rich, especially in the more prosperous states. And it is in more prosperous states that the intakes among the poor have declined relative to that found in less well off states such as Bihar, Orissa and West Bengal.

Trends in the iron gap and severity of deprivation indicated in Table 5.11 suggest that despite increased HCRs, depth and severity of iron deprivation has decreased for the poorest 25 per cent of the population at least among the poorer states. It is only the richest 25 per cent and the better off states that have seen worsening of the gap and severity of iron deprivation.

5.2.5 Vitamin C

In contrast to most nutrients, the principal sources of vitamin C in rural Indian diets are vegetables and fruits, and not cereals. The changes in dietary pattern outlined in section 5.1 highlighted the increased consumption of fruits and vegetables, and by larger numbers than before. Average vitamin C intakes have thus increased by 50 per cent from 40 mg to 61 mg per capita per day (Table 5.12). Correspondingly, the HCR of vitamin C deprivation decreased by nearly 25 percentage points between 1983 and 1999-2000. This increase in intakes may be seen in virtually all states; however, even so, HCRs exceed 50 per cent in states such as Andhra Pradesh, Kerala, Madhya Pradesh, Maharashtra and Rajasthan. There has also been a substantial fall in the depth and severity of vitamin C deprivation in all states (Table 5.13).

Intakes for the richest 25 per cent have increased more rapidly than among the poorest 25 per cent; thus, in most states there was a sharper decline in HCR among the richest as against the poorest. As far as gap and severity of the vitamin C deprivation is concerned, it is the poorest who have improved more than the rich as observed in Table 5.13.

Table 5.12

Average Vitamin C Intakes and Incidence of Vitamin C Deprivation, by Quartile Expenditure Group, between 1983 and 1999-2000

State	Vitamin C Intakes (mg per capita per day)						Incidence of Vitamin C Deprivation (%) (HCR)					
	1983			1999-2000			1983			1999-2000		
	Poorest 25%	Top 25%	All	Poorest 25%	Top 25%	All	Poorest 25%	Top 25%	All	Poorest 25%	Top 25%	All
Andhra Pradesh	18.6	45.9	29.5	32.2	66.6	48.3	94.8	61.7	81.2	77.7	21.5	52.9
Bihar	38.6	61.6	45.9	43.6	81.5	65.7	70.0	41.1	59.9	57.5	14.8	37.8
Gujarat	25.1	49.7	34.7	62.8	78.1	54.6	85.6	42.1	69.5	65.6	12.0	36.4
Haryana	28.0	62.3	39.0	33.1	76.4	58.8	78.5	41.8	67.4	75.0	13.2	39.1
Himachal Pradesh	25.1	54.6	37.2	29.9	69.7	52.6	82.2	48.1	68.9	81.6	21.6	51.0
Karnataka	17.8	43.0	28.8	28.9	68.2	48.0	95.5	55.4	79.8	80.7	29.6	56.9
Kerala	21.0	66.6	41.5	29.9	76.1	60.8	87.4	39.6	68.7	89.5	17.0	53.0
Madhya Pradesh	26.0	49.0	33.6	37.1	78.8	53.3	80.0	58.4	73.0	76.0	37.0	57.5
Maharashtra	19.0	42.2	29.0	31.5	65.3	46.1	92.7	58.2	78.8	80.4	20.0	51.8
Orissa	29.6	61.3	43.0	32.7	79.8	60.1	78.1	36.4	58.8	71.0	14.2	42.3
Punjab	32.2	69.5	48.7	40.1	118.2	77.5	68.6	35.6	53.0	60.2	8.7	31.0
Rajasthan	12.6	41.1	24.3	28.9	66.9	46.2	96.2	67.1	86.5	79.8	22.2	53.3
Tamil Nadu	15.4	47.9	27.3	29.5	65.9	48.8	96.3	58.6	83.6	81.6	21.9	50.8
Uttar Pradesh	24.6	65.1	41.8	49.4	92.4	72.6	82.9	41.6	64.2	63.6	16.7	39.6
West Bengal	39.1	100.2	60.7	69.6	105.9	87.4	64.3	15.1	41.8	43.1	6.7	22.5
Rural India	26.1	57.7	38.7	42.6	80.6	60.6	82.3	47.4	67.7	66.3	20.5	43.8

Source: Calculated from unit record data of the 38th and 55th NSSO rounds.

Table 5.13

Depth and Severity of Vitamin C Deprivation, by Quartile Expenditure Group, between 1983 and 1999-2000

State	Depth of Vitamin C Deprivation (FGT (1))						Severity of Vitamin C Deprivation (FGT(2))					
	1983			1999-2000			1983			1999-2000		
	Poorest 25%	Top 25%	All	Poorest 25%	Top 25%	All	Poorest 25%	Top 25%	All	Poorest 25%	Top 25%	All
Andhra Pradesh	0.56	0.25	0.40	0.29	0.05	0.16	0.37	0.13	0.24	0.14	0.02	0.07
Bihar	0.37	0.14	0.27	0.23	0.04	0.12	0.24	0.06	0.16	0.12	0.01	0.06
Gujarat	0.44	0.12	0.28	0.25	0.02	0.11	0.26	0.05	0.14	0.13	0.01	0.05
Haryana	0.48	0.15	0.33	0.29	0.03	0.12	0.34	0.07	0.20	0.14	0.01	0.05

contd...

...contd...

Himachal Pradesh	0.43	0.18	0.32	0.35	0.06	0.18	0.28	0.08	0.19	0.19	0.03	0.09
Karnataka	0.57	0.20	0.38	0.33	0.06	0.18	0.38	0.10	0.23	0.16	0.02	0.08
Kerala	0.60	0.13	0.38	0.41	0.04	0.19	0.45	0.06	0.25	0.23	0.01	0.09
Madhya Pradesh	0.50	0.24	0.38	0.38	0.12	0.24	0.36	0.13	0.25	0.24	0.05	0.13
Maharashtra	0.54	0.22	0.38	0.34	0.05	0.18	0.36	0.11	0.23	0.18	0.02	0.08
Orissa	0.41	0.13	0.26	0.31	0.03	0.15	0.27	0.06	0.15	0.17	0.01	0.07
Punjab	0.38	0.11	0.22	0.22	0.02	0.09	0.24	0.05	0.12	0.11	0.01	0.04
Rajasthan	0.71	0.31	0.52	0.36	0.06	0.19	0.55	0.18	0.36	0.20	0.02	0.09
Tamil Nadu	0.63	0.21	0.44	0.31	0.05	0.16	0.45	0.10	0.28	0.15	0.02	0.07
Uttar Pradesh	0.51	0.16	0.33	0.25	0.04	0.13	0.36	0.08	0.21	0.13	0.01	0.06
West Bengal	0.28	0.03	0.15	0.13	0.01	0.06	0.16	0.01	0.07	0.06	0.00	0.02
Rural India	0.48	0.18	0.33	0.27	0.05	0.15	0.33	0.09	0.20	0.14	0.02	0.07

Source: Calculated from unit record data of the 38th and 55th NSSO rounds

A closer examination of the vegetables and fruits food group indicates that the substantial increase in vitamin C over the period comes mainly from increased consumption of cabbage, potato, chili, cauliflower, guava and tomato as reported in Table 5.14. These items together account for 16 mg of the total 22 mg increase in per capita per day intakes of vitamin C.

Table 5.14

Per Capita Per Day Intake of Vitamin C (mg) from Vegetables and Fruits

Food item	*1983*	*1999-2000*
Potato	6.31	9.13
Cabbage	2.88	7.52
Chilli	2.62	4.8
Guava	2.74	4.75
Cauliflower	1.47	3.52
Tomato	1.17	3.12
Brinjal	1.42	1.57
Onion	0.81	1.23
Total	19.42	35.64

Source: Calculated from unit record data of the 38th and 55th NSSO rounds

5.2.6 Carotene (Vitamin A)

In the case of vitamin A as well, the principal source of the nutrient is not cereals but rather vegetables and fruits. These contribute almost half to vitamin A intake followed by animal products (milk and its products, meat, egg and fish) with a share of 23 per cent (Table 5.3). There are differences among states due in part to differences in food preferences. Milk is a major source of vitamin A in the northern states like Rajasthan, Haryana, Gujarat and Uttar Pradesh, while Karnataka, Andhra Pradesh, Tamil Nadu, West Bengal and Orissa have vegetables and fruits as their major source in 1999-2000. The milk share in total carotene intake is 45 per cent in Haryana as against 6 per cent for West Bengal in 1999-2000. In contrast, the vegetable and fruit share in total carotene is as high as 79 per cent in West Bengal as against 34 per cent for Haryana in 1999-2000. Similarly, meat, egg and fish have a higher share in total carotene intake in southern states as compared to northern states (Appendix Table A-5.1.3).

Despite diversification in the food basket towards vegetables, fruits and animal products, average intake of vitamin A declined in rural India from 1714 to 1651 μg. The HCR increased from 77.2 per cent to 78.6 per cent between 1983 and 1999-2000.

Of the total decline of 152 μg per day, 60 μg were accounted for by cereals and 80 μg by vegetables and fruits. Offsetting these, but only in part, was the increased consumption of milk and its products, meat, egg, etc., to the extent of 88 μg (Appendix Table A-5.1.4).

The decline in carotenoid intakes from fruits and vegetables merits closer scrutiny, as it appears contrary to expectations given the increased consumption of this commodity group. The detailed analysis at the item level in Table 5.15 reveals that intake of vitamin A from consumption of tomato, chilli, carrot, cabbage, potato, cauliflower, banana, orange, papaya has increased, while it has reduced from mango and green leafy vegetables between 1983 and 1999-2000.

Using the NSS data, we have found that the per capita consumption of green leafy vegetables has decreased from 30 g to 25 g per day between 1983 and 1999-2000. Various studies conducted by NNMB (1994-95) and others[6] have also found a reduction in the green leafy vegetables over time (Kumar and Mathur, 1996). And this has reduced overall contribution of vegetables and fruits. So it is the change in the composition of vegetables and fruits which has brought decrease in the intake of vitamin A.

6. For slum and rural communities in India, consumption of protective foods such as green leafy vegetables has declined over the years from 23 to 13 g per day, which is far below their RDA (Kumar and Mathur, 1996).

Table 5.15

Per Capita Per Day Intake of Vitamin A from Major Fruits and Vegetables

Vegetable and Fruit	*1983 (μg)*	*1999-2000 (μg)*
Tomato	15.3	40.6
Carrot	11.4	31.6
Chilli	4.2	15.5
Cabbage	2.8	7.3
Potato	8.9	12.9
Banana	3.4	6.5
Cauliflower	0.7	1.9
Pumpkin	1.7	2.8
Brinjal	8.7	9.7
Bitter gourd	1.3	1.9
Lady finger	2.0	2.5
Orange	3.9	4.2
Mango	124.0	87.1
Palak and other leafy vegetables	985.4	864.2

Source: Calculated from unit record data of the 38th and 55th NSSO rounds

Referring to Table 5.16, the average rural intake of vitamin A is much higher in Punjab, Haryana, West Bengal and Himachal Pradesh than Kerala, Tamil Nadu, Madhya Pradesh, Gujarat, Maharashtra and Andhra Pradesh. The prevalence of vitamin A deficiency (VAD) as measured by Bitot's spots, a clinical manifestation of VAD in the eye, reported in Table 5.17, also confirms this pattern to a large extent. The states of Haryana, Punjab, Himachal Pradesh show a much lower incidence of VAD than Tamil Nadu, Madhya Pradesh, Andhra Pradesh, Kerala, Gujarat, Maharashtra. The prevalence of VAD is typically much greater; data in support of this are however limited.

There is a mixed picture as far as pattern of change in the rural average intake of carotene for different states is concerned. Out of the 15 states considered, rural average intake of carotene has improved for Andhra Pradesh, Haryana, Karnataka, Kerala, Maharashtra, Rajasthan, Tamil Nadu, and Uttar Pradesh, while it has declined in Bihar, Gujarat, Madhya Pradesh, Orissa, Punjab, West Bengal, and Himachal Pradesh. Increases in average carotene intakes have translated into decreases in HCR except in Andhra Pradesh, and vice-versa.

Table 5.16

Average Vitamin A Intakes and Incidence of Vitamin A Deprivation, by Quartile Expenditure Group, between 1983 and 1999-2000

State	Intake of Vitamin A (µg per capita per day)						Incidence of Vitamin A Deprivation (%) (HCR)					
	1983			1999-2000			1983			1999-2000		
	Poorest 25%	Top 25%	All	Poorest 25%	Top 25%	All	Poorest 25%	Top 25%	All	Poorest 25%	Top 25%	All
Andhra Pradesh	902	2017	1389	1005	2144	1495	93.6	70.7	84.2	95.4	68.1	85.4
Bihar	2473	2441	2237	1160	2048	1460	65.9	67.8	69.8	84.0	68.2	78.7
Gujarat	1147	2295	1502	1023	2017	1417	92.2	66.4	85.3	94.5	73.9	88.4
Haryana	1529	3290	2197	1397	3576	2435	81.4	35.5	66.6	85.4	30.2	57.1
Himachal Pradesh	2124	3510	2674	1503	2781	1965	57.5	39.1	52.7	86.1	50.2	73.2
Karnataka	966	2080	1453	1235	2252	1744	94.1	67.0	82.5	85.5	61.3	75.8
Kerala	272	1360	693	487	1531	924	98.6	87.1	95.0	98.7	85.0	95.0
Madhya Pradesh	1556	2015	1630	1096	1976	1405	76.8	71.6	77.0	88.0	72.1	83.4
Maharashtra	899	1987	1345	1044	1994	1468	96.0	72.5	87.1	93.5	73.0	85.9
Orissa	2368	2435	2432	1517	2347	1917	64.1	58.2	62.3	78.1	62.4	72.5
Punjab	2022	4693	3182	1969	4554	3113	70.2	25.1	48.5	70.9	20.8	48.8
Rajasthan	931	2529	1568	953	2531	1657	92.9	63.7	82.7	95.7	58.1	79.9
Tamil Nadu	701	1490	986	751	1917	1323	95.8	83.4	92.2	98.6	73.7	88.2
Uttar Pradesh	778	2286	1395	916	2540	1563	90.5	64.8	81.3	90.7	60.3	78
West Bengal	2225	2886	2340	1851	2658	2123	64.8	46.9	60.1	73.6	51.8	65.3
Rural India	1341	2333	1713	1154	2394	1650	83.5	65.0	77.2	87.2	63.4	78.6

Table 5.17

Prevalence (%) of VAD

State/UT	Bitot's Spot (% of Population)
Andhra Pradesh	0.79
Bihar	0.14
Gujarat	0.20
Haryana	0.04
Himachal Pradesh	0.01
Karnataka	0.77
Kerala	0.25
Madhya Pradesh	2.62
Maharashtra	0.72
Orissa	0.86
Punjab	0.12
Rajasthan	0.22
Tamil Nadu	3.11
Pooled	0.21

Source: Department of Women and Child Development (1998). *India Nutrition Profile*. New Delhi: Ministry of Human Resource Development, Government of India.

Increase in carotene in these states has been mainly due to large increases in the intakes of the upper income groups. These increases have resulted in decreased HCRs, except in Andhra Pradesh.

The average carotene gap and severity of deprivation has worsened for the poorest 25 per cent of the population among the relatively poorer states of Bihar, Himachal Pradesh, Madhya Pradesh, Orissa and West Bengal. It is the richest 25 per cent of only Gujarat, Himachal Pradesh and Madhya Pradesh that have seen no improvement in depth and severity of carotene deprivation as evident in Table 5.18.

Table 5.18

Depth and Severity of Vitamin A Deprivation, by Quartile Expenditure Group, between 1983 and 1999-2000

	Depth of Vitamin A Deprivation (FGT (1))						*Severity of Vitamin A Deprivation (FGT(2))*					
	1983			*1999-2000*			*1983*			*1999-2000*		
State	*Poorest 25%*	*Top 25%*	*All*	*Poorest 25%*	*Top 25%*	*All*	*Poorest 25%*	*Top 25%*	*All*	*Poorest 25%*	*Top 25%*	*All*
Andhra Pradesh	0.63	0.36	0.5	0.56	0.24	0.41	0.47	0.22	0.34	0.37	0.12	0.24
Bihar	0.47	0.39	0.46	0.6	0.38	0.52	0.38	0.27	0.35	0.48	0.25	0.4
Gujarat	0.57	0.26	0.44	0.56	0.27	0.43	0.39	0.13	0.26	0.38	0.13	0.25
Haryana	0.51	0.11	0.32	0.43	0.09	0.23	0.35	0.05	0.19	0.26	0.04	0.12
Himachal Pradesh	0.31	0.12	0.23	0.49	0.17	0.34	0.2	0.05	0.13	0.33	0.08	0.19
Karnataka	0.59	0.3	0.45	0.52	0.24	0.37	0.41	0.17	0.30	0.36	0.12	0.23
Kerala	0.89	0.52	0.74	0.79	0.4	0.63	0.81	0.36	0.62	0.66	0.23	0.46
Madhya Pradesh	0.53	0.35	0.46	0.61	0.36	0.5	0.41	0.21	0.33	0.47	0.22	0.35
Maharashtra	0.62	0.35	0.49	0.55	0.28	0.42	0.44	0.21	0.33	0.37	0.14	0.25
Orissa	0.38	0.31	0.34	0.45	0.27	0.37	0.28	0.21	0.25	0.32	0.16	0.24
Punjab	0.39	0.06	0.2	0.31	0.04	0.16	0.24	0.03	0.11	0.17	0.01	0.08
Rajasthan	0.62	0.26	0.45	0.58	0.18	0.37	0.46	0.13	0.29	0.38	0.08	0.22
Tamil Nadu	0.7	0.46	0.61	0.67	0.3	0.49	0.55	0.30	0.45	0.49	0.15	0.32
Uttar Pradesh	0.71	0.32	0.54	0.65	0.27	0.47	0.6	0.20	0.41	0.51	0.15	0.33
West Bengal	0.34	0.21	0.29	0.38	0.21	0.31	0.24	0.12	0.19	0.24	0.11	0.2
Rural India	0.59	0.32	0.47	0.57	0.26	0.43	0.46	0.2	0.33	0.42	0.14	0.28

Source: Calculated from unit record data of the 38th and 55th NSSO rounds

5.2.7 Thiamine

As in case of calories and proteins, the major source of thiamine intake in rural India is cereals and pulses (Table 5.3). With declining share of cereals in the food basket, average rural intake of thiamine has decreased from 2.01 g to 1.79 g, translating into marginal increase in the incidence of thiamine deficiency from 9.1 to 9.7 per cent between 1983 and 1999-2000. Thus relative to other micronutrients, the magnitude of thiamine deficiency is relatively small.

Further, it appears to be a greater problem among populations consuming rice-based diets, although the evidence in Table 5.19 suggests that the average rural intake of thiamine for most of the states is much above the RDA of 1.2 mg. However, average intakes among the poorest 25 per cent of rice-eating states of Andhra Pradesh, Karnataka, Kerala, Orissa,

Table 5.19

Average Thiamine Intakes and Incidence of Thiamine Deprivation, by Quartile Expenditure Group, between 1983 and 1999-2000

State	*Thiamine Intakes (mg per capita per day)*						*Incidence of Thiamine Deprivation (%) (HCR)*					
	1983			*1999-2000*			*1983*			*1999-2000*		
	Poorest 25%	*Top 25%*	*All*	*Poorest 25%*	*Top 25%*	*All*	*Poorest 25%*	*Top 25%*	*All*	*Poorest 25%*	*Top 25%*	*All*
Andhra Pradesh	1.32	2.01	1.62	1.05	1.58	1.29	26.5	3.0	10.5	49.0	4.5	21.5
Bihar	1.64	2.79	2.19	1.46	2.28	1.85	11.3	0.1	3.7	11.5	0.3	3.7
Gujarat	1.53	2.43	1.92	1.45	2.01	1.69	10.4	1.1	4.0	10.0	1.0	3.9
Haryana	1.99	3.47	2.61	1.85	2.72	2.30	7.3	0.4	3.3	0.0	0.4	0.3
Himachal Pradesh	2.00	3.12	2.57	1.87	2.41	2.14	6.0	1.9	2.4	0.8	0.1	0.4
Karnataka	1.46	2.56	1.99	1.29	1.91	1.61	18.4	3.1	9.1	20.3	3.2	11.3
Kerala	0.71	1.62	1.11	0.85	1.56	1.21	91.2	7.9	47.1	77.8	5.9	35.5
Madhya Pradesh	1.72	2.97	2.22	1.43	2.44	1.91	14.3	0.1	4.7	21.6	1.0	7.9
Maharashtra	1.65	2.39	1.98	1.47	2.05	1.77	5.3	1.8	3.1	11.0	1.2	3.9
Orissa	1.01	2.00	1.47	1.09	1.80	1.42	52.2	0.9	16.3	31.9	0.2	10.2
Punjab	1.86	3.45	2.58	1.81	2.79	2.22	8.4	1.3	4.6	2.0	0.3	0.8
Rajasthan	2.15	3.60	2.79	2.11	3.06	2.55	3.5	0.6	1.8	2.0	0.3	0.4
Tamil Nadu	1.08	1.93	1.47	0.88	1.48	1.16	45.3	5.4	22.5	73.5	11.4	39.6
Uttar Pradesh	1.94	3.30	2.54	1.87	2.76	2.29	4.0	0.4	1.5	2.3	0.0	0.7
West Bengal	1.02	2.08	1.52	1.08	1.72	1.40	49.1	2.7	17.5	38.7	2.2	13.7
Rural India	1.56	2.58	2.01	1.43	2.17	1.79	20.3	2.5	9.1	21.0	2.9	9.7

Source: Calculated from unit record data of the 38th and 55th NSSO rounds

Tamil Nadu[7] and West Bengal are low, resulting in much higher rates of deprivation.[8]

Table 5.20

Depth and Severity of Thiamine Deprivation, by Quartile Expenditure Group, between 1983 and 1999-2000

State	Depth of Thiamine Deprivation (FGT (1))						Severity of Thiamine Deprivation (FGT(2))					
	1983			1999-2000			1983			1999-2000		
	Poorest 25%	Top 25%	All	Poorest 25%	Top 25%	All	Poorest 25%	Top 25%	All	Poorest 25%	Top 25%	All
Andhra Pradesh	0.05	0.006	0.02	0.08	0.004	0.03	0.018	0.002	0.007	0.022	0.001	0.007
Bihar	0.03	0.000	0.01	0.02	0.000	0.01	0.009	0.000	0.002	0.005	0.000	0.002
Gujarat	0.03	0.005	0.01	0.02	0.001	0.01	0.016	0.002	0.005	0.005	0.000	0.002
Haryana	0.03	0.000	0.01	0.00	0.000	0.00	0.021	0.000	0.008	0.000	0.000	0.000
Himachal Pradesh	0.03	0.005	0.01	0.00	0.000	0.00	0.020	0.001	0.006	0.000	0.000	0.000
Karnataka	0.05	0.007	0.02	0.04	0.004	0.02	0.022	0.003	0.008	0.010	0.001	0.005
Kerala	0.28	0.012	0.11	0.18	0.009	0.07	0.105	0.004	0.037	0.057	0.002	0.020
Madhya Pradesh	0.03	0.000	0.01	0.04	0.001	0.01	0.012	0.000	0.004	0.009	0.000	0.003
Maharashtra	0.01	0.003	0.01	0.02	0.002	0.01	0.005	0.001	0.002	0.008	0.001	0.003
Orissa	0.11	0.002	0.03	0.04	0.000	0.01	0.040	0.001	0.011	0.009	0.000	0.003
Punjab	0.04	0.004	0.02	0.00	0.001	0.00	0.026	0.002	0.012	0.001	0.001	0.001
Rajasthan	0.02	0.003	0.01	0.00	0.000	0.00	0.013	0.002	0.005	0.001	0.000	0.000
Tamil Nadu	0.13	0.006	0.05	0.16	0.013	0.07	0.054	0.001	0.017	0.046	0.003	0.018
Uttar Pradesh	0.01	0.001	0.00	0.01	0.000	0.00	0.007	0.000	0.002	0.003	0.000	0.001
West Bengal	0.12	0.004	0.04	0.06	0.002	0.02	0.048	0.001	0.015	0.017	0.000	0.005
Rural India	0.05	0.005	0.02	0.04	0.004	0.02	0.022	0.002	0.008	0.011	0.001	0.004

Source: Calculated from unit record data of the 38th and 55th NSSO rounds

Among the bottom 25 per cent of the population, the HCRs have increased for Andhra Pradesh, Karnataka, Tamil Nadu, Madhya Pradesh and Maharashtra, while decreased for Punjab, Haryana, Himachal Pradesh, Uttar Pradesh, Gujarat and Rajasthan. It is mainly Andhra Pradesh, Tamil Nadu and Maharashtra which have also worsened in terms of depth and severity of thiamine gap (Table 5.20).

7. Deficiency of thiamine is more common in certain parts of India, particularly in coastal districts of Andhra Pradesh since the diets consumed in these areas used to consist mainly of highly polished rice which is poor source of thiamine (Gopalan, 2000)
8. Top 25 per cent of population in states of Bihar, Gujarat, Haryana, Himachal Pradesh, Madhya Pradesh, Maharashtra, Orissa, Punjab, Rajasthan and Uttar Pradesh has less than one per cent thiamine deficiency.

5.2.8 Niacin

Cereals contribute the highest with 85 per cent of niacin intake (Table 5.3). Despite the decline in per capita cereal intake, the deficiency of niacin does not pose to be serious problem in rural India with only 15 per cent of the population being deficient.

It is cause of concern for states like Gujarat, Karnataka, Kerala, Maharashtra and Tamil Nadu, where more than half to one-third of the population is niacin-deficient (Table 5.21). This is well supported by the fact that in the Southern Peninsula of India, pellagra[9] has been observed in areas where *jowar*[10] is the main cereal consumed (Gopalan *et al.*, 2000). Further, for the poorest quartile in these states, the prevalence of inadequate niacin intakes ranges between 41 per cent to 78 per cent.

Table 5.21

Average Niacin Intakes and Incidence of Niacin Deprivation, by Quartile Expenditure Group, between 1983 and 1999-2000

State	*Niacin Intakes (per capita per day mg)*						*Incidence of Niacin Deprivation (%) (HCR)*					
	1983			*1999-2000*			*1983*			*1999-2000*		
	Poorest 25%	*Top 25%*	*All*	*Poorest 25%*	*Top 25%*	*All*	*Poorest 25%*	*Top 25%*	*All*	*Poorest 25%*	*Top 25%*	*All*
Andhra Pradesh	15.46	26.32	20.70	15.22	21.91	18.66	25.6	3.4	10.0	29.1	3.4	12.2
Bihar	14.18	29.83	21.89	16.60	24.32	20.43	39.5	1.0	12.5	15.8	2.0	6.5
Gujarat	11.44	20.40	15.60	11.35	17.46	14.15	73.3	12.2	37.7	78.2	21.6	48.5
Haryana	17.14	28.29	21.93	15.66	21.48	18.67	17.4	3.6	9.8	22.9	7.5	12.4
Himachal Pradesh	15.86	25.45	20.59	16.97	21.39	19.20	32.1	8.5	16.7	19.1	5.2	9.9
Karnataka	11.26	23.36	17.31	11.96	19.82	15.83	66.7	12.2	32.3	59.7	13.7	36.6
Kerala	10.86	21.46	15.69	12.88	20.23	16.73	76.8	7.1	37.6	56.2	8.4	25.1
Madhya Pradesh	16.46	29.24	22.59	15.06	23.11	19.27	18.5	2.6	7.6	29.7	4.6	13.8
Maharashtra	14.20	22.81	18.19	14.77	20.37	17.53	35.3	7.5	18.3	41.0	7.1	18.8
Orissa	14.50	29.43	21.93	16.71	25.51	21.40	30.1	1.8	8.8	10.3	0.5	3.3
Punjab	15.55	28.87	21.64	14.95	22.02	18.03	24.6	6.5	13.8	27.6	4.3	13.9
Rajasthan	12.70	28.96	20.84	16.00	23.97	19.65	39.6	5.2	17.9	31.6	6.2	16.7
Tamil Nadu	8.56	23.82	16.02	12.44	19.39	15.95	72.3	7.7	33.8	61.4	13.6	32.7
Uttar Pradesh	18.49	30.89	24.33	18.29	25.77	21.82	12.5	1.8	5.0	11.3	2.3	5.6
West Bengal	13.76	29.62	21.48	16.11	23.92	20.19	35.7	2.2	11.8	18.8	2.5	7.3
Rural India	15.34	26.80	20.87	16.15	21.83	19.17	33.1	5.5	15.3	25.2	8.2	14.8

Source: Calculated from unit record data of the 38th and 55th NSSO rounds

9. As noted in Chapter 3, pellagra is the disease caused by the deficiency of niacin. It is characterised by soreness of tongue, pigmented skin and diarrhoea.

10. Maize and *jowar* are poor sources of niacin.

Over time the HCR by quartile expenditure group of niacin deficiency has reduced for the poorest 25 per cent in relatively poor states of Bihar, West Bengal, Kerala, Orissa, Rajasthan, Tamil Nadu, Himachal Pradesh, Karnataka and Uttar Pradesh, and worsened in states of Andhra Pradesh, Gujarat, Haryana, Madhya Pradesh, Maharashtara and Punjab. As already pointed out in section 5.1, this pattern is because most of these poorer states had not experienced as sharp a fall in the cereal consumption as compared to richer states.

The depth and severity of the niacin deprivation has reduced for rural India as well as for bottom 25 per cent of the population in all states except for Madhya Pradesh and Maharashtra as evident in Table 5.22.

Table 5.22

Extent and Severity of Niacin Deprivation, by Quartile Expenditure Group, between 1983 and 1999-2000

	Extent of Niacin Deprivation						*Severity of Niacin Deprivation*					
	1983			*1999-2000*			*1983*			*1999-2000*		
State	*Poorest 25%*	*Top 25%*	*All*	*Poorest 25%*	*Top 25%*	*All*	*Poorest 25%*	*Top 25%*	*All*	*Poorest 25%*	*Top 25%*	*All*
Andhra Pradesh	0.052	0.009	0.022	0.041	0.004	0.016	0.020	0.005	0.010	0.013	0.001	0.005
Bihar	0.085	0.005	0.026	0.026	0.002	0.010	0.016	0.012	0.016	0.009	0.001	0.003
Gujarat	0.200	0.026	0.085	0.175	0.030	0.089	0.029	0.004	0.010	0.007	0.000	0.003
Haryana	0.070	0.012	0.032	0.027	0.008	0.014	0.082	0.011	0.033	0.056	0.007	0.025
Himachal Pradesh	0.091	0.034	0.046	0.031	0.004	0.014	0.046	0.007	0.019	0.005	0.001	0.002
Karnataka	0.208	0.028	0.085	0.154	0.020	0.081	0.046	0.022	0.023	0.007	0.001	0.003
Kerala	0.182	0.020	0.078	0.099	0.011	0.038	0.044	0.017	0.018	0.001	0.001	0.001
Madhya Pradesh	0.045	0.007	0.018	0.063	0.007	0.027	0.093	0.014	0.036	0.053	0.005	0.026
Maharashtra	0.064	0.019	0.032	0.073	0.009	0.028	0.064	0.013	0.027	0.028	0.003	0.010
Orissa	0.076	0.013	0.024	0.020	0.000	0.006	0.020	0.003	0.008	0.022	0.002	0.008
Punjab	0.078	0.025	0.047	0.038	0.007	0.019	0.022	0.011	0.012	0.024	0.002	0.008
Rajasthan	0.099	0.018	0.043	0.069	0.007	0.031	0.031	0.010	0.011	0.008	0.000	0.002
Tamil Nadu	0.229	0.020	0.087	0.119	0.016	0.056	0.047	0.014	0.028	0.009	0.002	0.005
Uttar Pradesh	0.031	0.005	0.012	0.020	0.003	0.009	0.040	0.011	0.018	0.021	0.001	0.008
West Bengal	0.102	0.008	0.034	0.031	0.004	0.011	0.102	0.012	0.036	0.034	0.004	0.015
Rural India	0.086	0.016	0.037	0.049	0.012	0.025	0.014	0.003	0.006	0.007	0.001	0.003

Source: Calculated from unit record data of the 38th and 55th NSSO rounds

5.2.9 Riboflavin

Unlike the other vitamins of vitamin-B group, the prevalence of riboflavin inadequacy is high at 61 per cent in 1983 and it further increases to 67 per cent in 1999-2000 for rural India. It is important to note that milk and milk products, meat, egg, fish and green vegetables are also good sources of riboflavin besides cereals[11] and pulses (Table 5.3).

Some of the prosperous states like Punjab and Haryana have 40 per cent of population deficient in riboflavin intake, while poorer states like Orissa and West Bengal have more than 75 per cent of population deficient in riboflavin intake. Inadequacy is greater among the poorest quartile, averaging around 80 per cent for Punjab and Haryana and more than 90 per cent for poorest in other states in 1999-2000.

Between 1983 and 1999-2000, we have two important observations (Table 5.23). First, increase in riboflavin deficiency in the bottom 25 per cent of the population is much more in richer states of Punjab, Haryana and Himachal Pradesh than poorer states of Bihar, Orissa, West Bengal, Madhya Pradesh, etc. Secondly, increase in riboflavin deficiency in top 25 per cent of the population is much more for the relatively poorer states of Bihar, Orissa and West Bengal than richer states of Haryana and Himachal Pradesh. This kind of trend is the direct outcome of dietary changes taking place. Cereal consumption has not fallen for the bottom 25 per cent of the population in poorer states as against relatively prosperous states. Further, the fall in the cereal intakes of the top 25 per cent has been compensated by non-cereal food more in richer states, especially Punjab, than relatively poorer states.

Among the poorest 25 per cent, it is mainly in states of Andhra Pradesh, Gujarat, Karnataka, Madhya Pradesh and Tamil Nadu which have deteriorated in terms of depth and severity of the gap of riboflavin deficiency over 1983 and 1999-2000 (Table 5.24). As far as top 25 per cent of the population is concerned, depth and severity of the riboflavin gap has increased in most of the states except Andhra Pradesh, Himachal Pradesh, Kerala, Punjab and Rajasthan.

---

11. Rice is a poor source of riboflavin.

Table 5.23

Average Riboflavin Intakes and Incidence of Riboflavin Deprivation, by Quartile Expenditure Group, between 1983 and 1999-2000

	Riboflavin Intakes (mg per capita per day)						*Incidence of Riboflavin Deprivation (%) (HCR)*					
	1983			*1999-2000*			*1983*			*1999-2000*		
State	*Poorest 25%*	*Top 25%*	*All*	*Poorest 25%*	*Top 25%*	*All*	*Poorest 25%*	*Top 25%*	*All*	*Poorest 25%*	*Top 25%*	*All*
Andhra Pradesh	0.84	1.53	1.14	0.81	1.41	1.08	90.3	29.1	61.9	96.9	36.3	72.9
Bihar	0.81	2.32	1.45	0.79	1.39	1.06	91.9	20.9	62.4	97.0	32.0	70.4
Gujarat	0.94	1.64	1.26	0.89	1.46	1.13	80.4	21.9	48.7	92.0	33.8	66.2
Haryana	1.01	2.22	1.53	0.99	2.13	1.56	73.9	5.4	35.5	80.5	14.2	38.2
Himachal Pradesh	0.94	1.82	1.34	1.16	1.66	1.41	75.9	16.1	42.2	86.6	19.4	50.9
Karnataka	0.74	1.71	1.17	0.74	1.44	1.08	94.3	27.5	62.9	98.2	42.2	76.1
Kerala	0.87	2.07	1.42	0.70	1.46	1.06	93.9	41.1	75.7	98.8	34.5	72.5
Madhya Pradesh	0.79	1.65	1.18	0.75	1.43	1.06	94.1	22.0	61.2	98.0	37.9	74.6
Maharashtra	0.76	1.32	1.01	0.77	1.31	1.02	93.7	49.4	75.4	95.7	55.6	78.8
Orissa	0.75	1.66	1.14	0.81	1.32	1.06	97.0	27.8	69.6	96.8	42.9	76.2
Punjab	0.95	2.13	1.50	1.00	2.15	1.48	75.1	9.3	35.4	82.3	6.6	39.9
Rajasthan	0.99	2.14	1.53	1.03	2.03	1.52	69.1	10.0	36.5	67.9	7.4	32.9
Tamil Nadu	0.65	1.49	1.02	0.67	1.27	0.95	95.3	39.7	74.1	99.5	50.5	82.3
Uttar Pradesh	0.84	1.78	1.26	0.90	1.66	1.24	90.5	16.8	53.3	89.5	20.4	56.1
West Bengal	0.77	2.02	1.32	0.82	1.31	1.05	93.8	36.6	71.9	95.8	45.6	76.2
Rural India	0.81	1.81	1.26	0.83	1.53	1.14	90.7	27.2	61.0	94.2	34.1	67.2

Source: Calculated from unit record data of the 38th and 55th NSSO rounds

5.3 Bioavailability of Nutrients in Rural Indian Diet

Till now the focus of the study has been to quantify nutrient deficiencies in terms of nutrient intakes. However, in determining the nutritional status, what is crucial is the absorption of nutrient intakes or bioavailability of the nutrient rather than the amount of nutrient ingested. But there is no simple scientific way to calculate quantitatively how much of each known nutrient intake is being absorbed from the diet, as it involves complex interactions inside the body.

Table 5.24

Depth and Severity of Riboflavin Deprivation, by Expenditure Quartile Group, between 1983 and 1999-2000

State	*Extent of Riboflavin Deprivation (FGT (1))*						*Severity of Riboflavin Deprivation (FGT(2))*					
	1983			*1999-2000*			*1983*			*1999-2000*		
	Poorest 25%	*Top 25%*	*All*	*Poorest 25%*	*Top 25%*	*All*	*Poorest 25%*	*Top 25%*	*All*	*Poorest 25%*	*Top 25%*	*All*
Andhra Pradesh	0.29	0.05	0.15	0.32	0.05	0.19	0.115	0.013	0.051	0.125	0.011	0.068
Bihar	0.35	0.03	0.17	0.32	0.05	0.18	0.160	0.007	0.063	0.126	0.010	0.068
Gujarat	0.27	0.04	0.13	0.33	0.06	0.19	0.119	0.014	0.050	0.141	0.015	0.078
Haryana	0.17	0.01	0.08	0.20	0.02	0.11	0.064	0.002	0.026	0.062	0.006	0.034
Himachal Pradesh	0.22	0.03	0.10	0.20	0.02	0.11	0.089	0.008	0.035	0.061	0.004	0.033
Karnataka	0.36	0.05	0.18	0.36	0.07	0.21	0.166	0.016	0.070	0.156	0.016	0.086
Kerala	0.48	0.08	0.27	0.42	0.05	0.24	0.264	0.022	0.123	0.198	0.014	0.106
Madhya Pradesh	0.32	0.03	0.15	0.37	0.06	0.22	0.131	0.007	0.052	0.159	0.016	0.087
Maharashtra	0.34	0.09	0.21	0.35	0.10	0.23	0.147	0.027	0.078	0.149	0.027	0.088
Orissa	0.37	0.03	0.18	0.29	0.06	0.18	0.163	0.008	0.064	0.106	0.012	0.059
Punjab	0.22	0.01	0.09	0.18	0.01	0.10	0.088	0.004	0.032	0.058	0.002	0.030
Rajasthan	0.22	0.02	0.09	0.17	0.01	0.09	0.094	0.006	0.036	0.056	0.002	0.029
Tamil Nadu	0.44	0.08	0.24	0.43	0.09	0.26	0.231	0.022	0.103	0.200	0.026	0.113
Uttar Pradesh	0.28	0.03	0.13	0.25	0.03	0.14	0.114	0.006	0.045	0.090	0.007	0.048
West Bengal	0.42	0.06	0.22	0.33	0.07	0.20	0.219	0.016	0.091	0.130	0.017	0.073
Rural India	0.33	0.05	0.17	0.31	0.06	0.17	0.147	0.014	0.063	0.123	0.015	0.057

Source: Calculated from unit record data of the 38th and 55th NSSO rounds

Some recent studies (Bhargava *et al.*, 2001; Tseng *et al.*, 1997) have taken up issue of bioavailability specifically with regard to iron intakes. They have attempted to estimate the bioavailable iron from mixed diets, taking into account the enhancers and inhibitors of iron absorption under alternative assumptions on body iron stores as discussed in section 3.5.4.

Using information from 24-hour dietary recall data and allowing for nutrient interactions at each meal, these studies have calculated bioavailable iron by computing intakes of dietary iron, iron from animal sources, ascorbic acid, phytates and tannins. Their results show poor diet quality which is primarily based on cereal, and has low intake of vitamins which is an important factor that contributes to iron deficiency anaemia.

One limitation of NSS data set is that it does not allow us to discuss factors of human physiology, factors specific to health status and factors related to the food processing in determining the bioavailability of nutrients. However, we provide some evidence on the bioavailability which may have resulted from the changes in diet quality that have been observed in rural India between 1983 and 1999-2000.

It is well known that a more balanced diet has a significant beneficial impact on bioavailability of the nutrients. Over time, as demonstrated above, dietary composition has shifted from cereals to non-cereals and there has been an increase in the intake of vitamin C and fat for all quartiles among all states in rural India. This is significant, as both vitamin C and fat are important in enhancing the bioavailability of many micronutrients. For example, an increase in the intake of vitamin C acts as enhancer in the absorption of iron (Gopalan *et al.*, 2000).

Table 5.25 suggests that between 1983 and 1999-2000: (i) intake of vitamin C has increased by 22 mg, and (ii) consumption of meat, fish and poultry has also increased from 9.6 g to 12.03 g. These two factors have increased the enhancing factor defined in section 3.5.4 from 48.39 to 72.97. This would increase the absorption of iron as set out there and as suggested by Bhargava *et al.* (2001). This may result in lower prevalence of iron deficiency in India than indicated by the calculations based on iron intakes alone.

Table 5.25

Variables Used for Calculating Bioavailable Iron

Variable	*1983*	*1999-2000*
MFP (gm) (Meat, fish, poultry)	9.6	12.03
Vitamin C (mg)	38.79	60.93
EF=MFP+VIT C	48.39	72.97

Source: Calculated from unit record data of the 38th and 55th NSSO rounds

Similarly, an increase in the consumption of fat of 10 mg in rural Indian population would improve the absorption of vitamin A. Not considering the effect of increase in the fat intake may mean overestimation of the trends in vitamin A deprivation. Similarly, the presence of fat in the diet reduces the need for thiamine; therefore, taking into account this role would definitely reduce level of thiamine deficiency, which is a matter of concern at the lower end of the income spectrum, as well as affect the trend in thiamine deficiency.

There are limitations to such adjustments for bioavailability as these demand detailed individual-level information cannot be implemented using data on consumption during the last 30 days.

5.4 Summarising the Nutritional Outcomes across States

This section now reviews the evidence on nutritional outcomes based on data from the 1998-99 demographic and health survey for India. Consider first, the percentage of women whose body mass index (BMI) is below 18.5 (Table 5.26). Punjab and Haryana have the lowest percentage of underweight women, while Bihar, Madhya Pradesh, Rajasthan and Uttar Pradesh (BIMARU) states have nearly half the women being undernourished.

Table 5.26

Level of Nutrient Intakes and Nutritional Status of the Population in Rural India, 1999-2000

State	*Per Capita Calorie Intake (kcal)*	*Per Capita Iron Intake (mg)*	*% of Women having BMI<18.5*	*% of Children having weight-for-age below minus 2SD*	*% of Women having*			*% of Children having*		
					Moderate Anaemia	*Severe Anaemia*	*Anaemia of any kind*	*Moderate Anaemia*	*Severe Anaemia*	*Anaemia of any kind*
Andhra Pradesh	2029	19.54	43.5	40.7	15.32	2.59	50.7	45.45	5.06	73.5
Bihar	2116	24.67	40.6	55.1	19.08	1.45	64.0	50.55	3.92	81.4
Gujarat	2004	23.42	48.8	49.3	16.78	3.10	51.4	47.88	8.43	79.1
Haryana	2460	24.70	31.3	35.5	16.12	1.65	47.5	59.45	7.10	82.9
Himachal Pradesh	2460	22.93	31.3	44.9	7.06	0.14	43.1	42.64	2.97	62.8
Karnataka	2029	20.79	47.8	46.4	8.40	0.70	46.2	45.12	7.05	72.3
Kerala	2006	19.96	20.3	28.0	15.35	2.85	23.5	19.06	0.50	43.2
Madhya Pradesh	2059	22.62	40.4	58.4	2.62	0.52	57.0	49.54	4.39	75.4
Maharashtra	2020	22.29	50.2	53.2	16.89	1.01	50.6	50.83	3.53	77.9
Orissa	2142	23.46	50.4	55.5	14.30	2.51	64.3	43.42	3.07	72.7
Punjab	2393	24.65	20.7	31.9	16.39	1.57	42.5	57.17	7.06	80.8
Rajasthan	2423	29.37	39.4	51.9	13.40	0.81	49.1	52.85	9.08	82.3
Tamil Nadu	1836	17.79	35.9	38.4	13.81	1.72	58.6	42.58	6.46	70.2
Uttar Pradesh	2331	26.61	50.9	52.7	17.68	3.19	64.1	49.99	2.85	80.7
West Bengal	2107	23.00	39.8	53.6	16.61	1.39	49.5	48.99	6.94	73.3
Rural India	2145	23.04	41.0	49.6	13.64	1.66	53.9	45.31	4.74	74.9

Source: Calculated from NSS (1999-2000) round and NFHS (1998-99) survey.

Preschool children constitute the other most nutritionally vulnerable group; their nutritional status is considered to be a sensitive indicator of community health and nutrition. A similar picture appears to characterise underweight children. Thus, this anthropometric measure of adverse nutritional status appears to be correlated with poverty at the state level.

The same cannot be said, however, for other indicators of malnutrition. For example, the Demographic and Health Survey (DHS) data also contain information on anaemia which is related to insufficient intake of dietary iron. When all categories of anaemia (mild, moderate and severe) are considered, the prevalence of anaemia among children is high not only in Bihar and Rajasthan, but also as high as 80 per cent in the prosperous states of Haryana and Punjab. It is relatively low in states such as Kerala. When the prevalence of moderate and severe anemia is examined separately, these four states again have high incidence of moderate and severe anaemia among children as compared to other states. More than half of children are moderately anaemic in Bihar, Haryana, Punjab and Rajasthan as against only 19 per cent in Kerala.

Similarly, prevalence of anemia of any kind among women is not only as high as 64 per cent in Bihar, Orissa and West Bengal, but it is also more than 40 per cent for relatively prosperous states like Gujarat, Haryana, Punjab, etc. The scenario remains the same even when we observe the prevalence of moderate and severe anemia separately.

5.5 Relating Nutrient Intakes to Nutritional Outcomes

Inadequate nutrition is a problem throughout India. However, observing Table 5.26, we find that there is no obvious relationship between the level of nutrient intake and nutritional status of the population.

At first glance, there appears to be little relationship between the ranking of states by nutritional status and that by nutrient intakes. Anthropometric indicators for women and preschool children are worse in states like Bihar, Orissa and Uttar Pradesh as compared to states like Kerala and Tamil Nadu despite lower levels of calorie and micronutrient intake in the latter. Bihar, Orissa and Uttar Pradesh have high energy intakes with more than 2,100 kcal as average per capita per day calorie intake, but at the same time, more than 40 per cent of women have BMI less than 18.5. The average per capita per day energy intake of Tamil Nadu is more than 250 kcal lower than these states but prevalence of underweight among women is 36 per cent.

Similarly, in comparing iron intakes with anemic status of the population, there appears to be no one-to-one relationship. The average per capita per day iron intake in Bihar, Haryana, Punjab and Rajasthan is above the RDA of 24 mg. Nevertheless, 40-60 per cent of the women are anaemic and 60-80 per cent of the preschool children are anaemic. The iron intake in Kerala is lower than the RDA, yet it does not have a high prevalence of anaemia among women and preschool children. In Kerala, only 23 per cent of women and 43 per cent of preschool children are suffering from anaemia of any kind.

According to Prema Ramchandran (2004), despite low level of nutrient intake, the undernutrition rates in Tamil Nadu, Andhra Pradesh and Gujarat are low because of well organised food supplementation through Integrated Child Development Scheme (ICDS). Similarly, according to NFHS (1998-99), low rates of undernutrition in children in Kerala and Tamil Nadu as compared to Maharashtra and Gujarat is the result of appropriate infant and child feeding practices, habits, better access to health care for children, and more equitable distribution of food within family and state.

According to the NFHS (1998-99), infection contributes significantly to anaemia in rural India. Infection in turn is related to poor sanitation, non-availability of safe drinking water and poor hygiene and caring practices of the population.

Thus, in general, nutrient intake is only one of the factors that determines the nutritional status of the population. Nutritional status is the outcome of the interplay of complex, multidimensional factors. In other words, to determine the nutritional status of the population, one needs to go beyond the simple measure of assessing the nutrient intakes which have been analysed in chapter 7.

The summary statistics of these socioeconomic and environmental variables is discussed in Appendix A-5.2.

5.6 A Summary of the Evidence

The principal contribution of this part of the research work is to document, perhaps systematically for the first time, the magnitude of nutrient deprivation, especially micronutrient deprivation in rural diets in India, and how this has changed over a period of time with dietary changes between 1983 and 1999-2000.

In rural India, there has been dietary diversification as indicated from the declining share of cereals in total food expenditure and increasing share of milk, meat, vegetables and fruits over time. This substitution has not only occurred among the richest but also among the poorest, though the change is much more profound for the rich than the poor. This shift in the tastes has led to decline of almost 2 kg in per capita per month cereal consumption between 1983 and 1999-2000 in rural India. However, the magnitude of decline varies from only 300 g for the poorest to around 4 kg for the richest population of rural India. It is this poorest section of the population which influences the state-level outcomes of nutrient intakes. The increase in the cereal intake of the poorest in states of Kerala, Orissa, West Bengal and Bihar explain the lowest decline of around ½ kg as compared to richer states of Haryana and Punjab which have a substantial decline of 3 kg mainly as these experience the contrary.

Similarly, doubling of the number of commodities consumed led to an increase in the value of DDI indicative of diet diversification.

Despite the unambiguous evidence of diversification in terms of increased number of households, it is important to note that a fairly high percentage of sample households—about one-third—report no consumption of fluid milk or of fruits. Thus, there are still large numbers of people who do not consume the 'higher-quality' foods and are responsible for high levels of nutrient deprivation.

Trends in nutrient adequacy do not portray a very encouraging picture for rural India. It is a matter of concern that among nutrients, average intakes were at or above the RDA only for protein, thiamine, vitamin C and niacin, but below the RDA for calories, fat, riboflavin, iron and vitamin A in 1999-2000. Three-fourths of rural Indians have dietary intakes of vitamin A and iron below the RDA; nearly two-thirds have below-RDA intakes of riboflavin; nearly half of population was deficient in calorie intakes; and around 38 per cent are not getting the minimum required protein intakes. Further, despite improvements in the availability of vitamin C and fat, HCRs of nutrient deprivation are as high as 44 per cent and 64 per cent respectively. It is only in the case of thiamine and niacin that the head count percentage of deprivation is relatively low, at about 10 per cent and 15 per cent respectively. Not surprisingly, deprivation levels are much higher among the poor than among the rich.

In general, states of Haryana, Himachal Pradesh, Rajasthan, Punjab, and Uttar Pradesh perform much better in most of the nutrient intakes than states of Andhra Pradesh, Gujarat, Karnataka, Kerala, Maharashtra, Tamil Nadu, Bihar, Madhya Pradesh, Orissa and West Bengal.

The pattern of changes in intake of vitamin C and fat are distinct from those in the other seven nutrients. With dietary diversification, there has been substantial increase in the average intake of vitamin C and fat for rural India along with decrease in HCR, and depth and severity of nutrient gap over time. This has been unambiguously experienced for all states, both on an average as well as different quartile levels. However, the average intake of other seven nutrients has decreased in rural India between 1983 and 1999-2000. And it has correspondingly translated into increased HCRs. However, depth and severity of the nutrient gap has decreased for all nutrients except iron. This trend of declining calorie and protein intakes is in line with the results of Meenakshi and Vishwanathan (2001) and Shariff and Mallick (2001), who studied the trend till 1993-94. Shariff and Mallick (2001) also suggest an increase in iron deficiency.

The poorest quartile saw an increase in the incidence of the deficiency for all nutrients except niacin[12]; however, the depth and severity of the gap has decreased in all cases.

What is surprising is that nutrient deprivation has increased over time, not just among the poor, but also among the richest 25 per cent, except vitamin A where deprivation for the richest has not increased.

Broadly speaking, there has been an increase in the incidence of deficiency levels of these nutrients in most of the states[13] with few exceptions. The incidence of calorie deficiency has not increased only in states of Kerala, West Bengal and Orissa. The percentage of population

12. Marginal improvements in the intake of calorie, riboflavin and niacin have resulted in decrease in incidence of deprivation for niacin only.

13. Except protein, Kerala experiences fall in HCR for all the eight nutrients considered. Interestingly, even after decrease, these levels remain among the highest in rural India.

getting less than minimum required protein, riboflavin and iron has increased in all states except for Rajasthan in case of protein, and Kerala in case of riboflavin and iron. Andhra Pradesh, Madhya Pradesh, Karnataka, Maharashtra and Tamil Nadu are some states which have experienced increase in HCRs for thiamine intakes as against the decline in rest of the states. The evidence for niacin and vitamin A are mixed with half of states witnessing increase in the level of deficiency and other half witnessing a decline.

This pattern is true for the poorest quartile as well. Except for vitamin C and fat, there has been increase in the incidence of nutrient deprivation in most of the states. However, the poor among the poorer states of Kerala, West Bengal, Orissa and Bihar experienced a decline in HCR of nutrient deprivation except vitamin A (not primarily sourced in cereals).

Given the overwhelming evidence of diversification in the dietary basket of goods over time, it is somewhat paradoxical to observe that level of deprivation has not decreased for most of the nutrients (with the exception of fat and vitamin C) in most of the states, both on average and at quartile levels. Diversification in the dietary intake has implied lower cereal intakes, a decline which explains virtually all of the decreased nutrient intakes observed as it accounts for almost three-fourths of these nutrient intakes except vitamin A. While there has been increased consumption of other commodities such as vegetables, fruits, milk, meat and so on, these have not been of sufficiently high orders of magnitude to offset the consequences of reduced cereal intakes. Therefore, bottom 25 per cent of poorer states which experience no fall or minimal decrease in their cereal intake have not worsened in the terms of these nutrient intakes. As far as vitamin A is concerned, though it is primarily sourced in vegetables and fruits, its intake has decreased primarily on account of change in composition of vegetables and fruits, especially the apparent decrease in consumption of green leafy vegetables.

These interpretations need to be qualified in light of issues associated with nutrient norms as discussed in section 4.1.

In general, the higher nutrient intake of the northern states does not signify better nutritional status of the northern states as compared to the southern states. Besides age, sex and physical activity status, there are many factors that determine the average intakes of the population like climatological factors, behavioural factors, cultural factors and overall physical environment. It can be argued that if one takes into account differences in climate, dietary habits, water, sanitation facilities and health care facilities existing in the southern states as compared to northern states, then these differences in the average nutrient intakes may not seem realistic.

Further, we are assuming nutrient ingested is actually absorbed by the body which does not distinguish between bioavailability of nutrients from availability of the nutrients. For example, regions with better water and sanitation facilities would require less nutrient on two fronts—lower loss and lower nutrient requirement to fight against the water-borne diseases and better absorption as compared to regions without it (Scrimshaw *et al.*, 1959).

Bringing in this concept of absorption or utilisation of nutrients can probably provide a possible explanation for better anthropometric status in southern states of Kerala, Tamil Nadu and Karnataka, besides ranking low in relation to other Indian states in terms of average nutrient intakes.

The diversification in the diet from cereals to non-cereals among all income groups in rural India, that is, increased consumption of milk, meat, egg, etc., would imply improved quality of protein which should mean lowering of the protein requirement as discussed by a nutritionist. Thus, lowering of the RDA of protein would lower the estimates of the protein deprivation.

With increased mechanisation and fewer hours of work, there is need to revise the calorie norm downwards from the present level of 2,400 kcal. Any downward change in the norm would seriously affect the calorie deprivation figures and may even provide reconciliation between income-based and calorie-based poverty estimates.

Keeping in mind the above facts, it may be possible that levels of deprivation may scale down or trend of worsening nutrient intakes may no longer hold. But the fact that a sizeable proportion of rural Indian population is deficient in most of the nutrients would still stand. While income and deprivation are certainly correlated, malnutrition appears not to afflict the poor alone.

The evidence on nutritional status indicates that it is not only the BIMARU states of rural India which have high prevalence of underweight and anaemia among women and children but also relatively richer states like Punjab and Haryana which otherwise have high intake of nutrients. Further, states like Kerala and Tamil Nadu which do not rank high in terms of nutrient intakes certainly perform better in terms of nutritional status. It supports that nutrient intake is only one of the crucial factors that influences nutritional status.

Therefore, to understand the possible reasons for variations in the nutrient intakes and nutritional status, we estimate nutrient demand functions and study the determinants of nutritional status in Chapter 6 and Chapter 7 respectively. Nutrient demand functions are estimated by operating in the nutrient space rather than commodity space, following the work of Lancaster (1971). This exercise focuses on the role of income, occupational structure, social status, seasonality, education and head of the household in determining the demand for these nutrients. Similarly, nutritional status is estimated as a health production function with nutrient intakes and non-nutrient factors as inputs. The results of these exercises have implications for effective targetting and design of policy interventions to alleviate micronutrient malnutrition.

Appendix Table A-5.1.1

Contribution (%) of Various Foods to Nutrient Intakes, by Quartile Expenditure Group, in 1983 and 1999-2000

	Calories										Protein									
	1999-2000					1983					1999-2000					1983				
Food group	Q1	Q2	Q3	Q4	All	Q1	Q2	Q3	Q4	All	Q1	Q2	Q3	Q4	All	Q1	Q2	Q3	Q4	All
Cereals	77	72	67	59	69	83	79	75	66	76	77	72	67	59	69	80	76	72	64	73
Pulses	4	4	5	5	4	4	4	5	5	5	9	10	11	12	11	8	10	11	12	10
Milk and milk products	2	4	6	11	6	2	3	5	8	5	3	6	9	14	8	2	5	7	11	6
Meat, egg and fish	1	1	1	1	1	0	1	1	1	1	3	4	4	5	4	2	3	4	5	4
Vegetables and fruits	6	6	6	7	6	4	4	4	5	4	6	6	7	7	6	5	4	4	5	4
Oils	6	6	7	8	7	3	3	4	5	4	0	0	0	0	0	0	0	0	0	0
Other food	5	6	8	10	7	5	6	7	10	7	2	2	2	3	2	2	2	3	3	3
	Fat										Vitamin C									
	1999-2000					1983					1999-2000					1983				
Food group	Q1	Q2	Q3	Q4	All	Q1	Q2	Q3	Q4	All	Q1	Q2	Q3	Q4	All	Q1	Q2	Q3	Q4	All
Cereals	24	19	15	11	17	44	33	26	19	30	0.2	0	0	1	0.4	1	1	1	1	1
Pulses	2	2	2	2	2	3	2	3	3	3	0.1	0	0	0	0.1	1	0	0	1	1
Milk and milk products	10	17	24	33	21	9	16	22	30	19	1.9	3	5	7	4.3	3	4	6	8	5
Mea, egg and fish	2	2	2	2	2	1	2	2	2	2	0.3	0	0	0	0.3	0	0	0	0	0
Vegetables and fruits	4	5	6	7	5	5	5	6	7	5	94	92	90	88	91	84	85	84	82	84
Oils	54	52	48	42	49	34	37	37	35	36	0	0	0	0	0	0	0	0	0	0
Other food	3	3	3	4	4	5	5	5	5	5	4	4	4	4	3.9	10	9	8	8	9

contd...

...contd...

Food group	Vitamin A										Niacin									
	1999-2000					1983					1999-2000					1983				
	Q1	Q2	Q3	Q4	All	Q1	Q2	Q3	Q4	All	Q1	Q2	Q3	Q4	All	Q1	Q2	Q3	Q4	All
Cereals	14	11	9	6	10	25	19	15	11	17	89	88	86	82	86	88	88	86	83	86
Pulses	5	5	4	3	4	5	5	5	4	5	3.2	4	4	5	3.8	3	3	4	5	4
Milk and milk products	10	16	22	29	19	7	13	19	25	16	0.3	0	1	1	0.7	0	0	1	1	0
Meat, egg and fish	2	3	3	4	3	1	1	1	2	1	0.5	1	1	1	0.7	0	0	1	1	1
Vegetables and fruits	62	57	54	49	56	52	51	49	45	49	5.1	6	7	8	6.4	6	6	6	7	6
Oils	1	2	3	4	2	1	2	2	4	2	0	0	0	0	0.1	0	0	0	0	0
Other food	6	5	6	6	6	9	9	8	8	9	1.7	2	2	3	2.2	2	2	2	3	2

Food group	Thiamine										Iron									
	1999-2000					1983					1999-2000					1983				
	Q1	Q2	Q3	Q4	All	Q1	Q2	Q3	Q4	All	Q1	Q2	Q3	Q4	All	Q1	Q2	Q3	Q4	All
Cereals	82	79	76	71	77	78	75	70	62	71	78	76	74	70	74	79	78	77	72	76
Pulses	6	7	7	8	7	4	5	5	6	5	5	5	6	6	5	4	5	5	6	5
Milk and milk products	1	2	3	6	3	4	7	11	17	10	1	1	1	2	1	0	1	1	2	1
Meat, egg and fish	1	1	1	1	1	0	0	1	1	0	1	1	1	2	1	1	1	1	1	1
Vegetables and fruits	9	9	10	11	10	10	10	10	11	10	9	10	11	12	10	10	8	8	9	9
Oils	0	0	0	0	0	0	0	0	0	0	0	0	0	0	0	0	0	0	0	0
Other food	1.79	2	2.4	3.3	2	3	3	3	4	3	6	7	7	8	7	6	7	7	9	7

Food group	Riboflavin									
	1999-2000					1983				
	Q1	Q2	Q3	Q4	All	Q1	Q2	Q3	Q4	All
Cereals	74	68	62	52	64	86	84	81	76	82
Pulses	4	5	5	5	5	5	6	7	8	7
Milk and milk products	6	11	16	25	15	1	2	2	4	2
Meat, egg and fish	1	2	2	2	2	0	0	0	1	0
Vegetables and fruits	12	12	12	12	12	5	6	6	8	6
Oils	0	0	0	0	0	0	0	0	0	0
Other food	2	2	3	3	3	2	2	3	4	3

Note: Q1, Q2, Q3 and Q4 refer to poorest, second, third and top expenditure quartile group

Source: Calculated from unit record data of the 38th and 55th NSSO rounds

Appendix Table A-5.1.2

Absolute Protein Intake (g) from Different Food Groups

Food Group	*1983*	*1999-2000*
Cereal	46.8	40.1
Pulses	6.9	6.5
Milk and its products	5.0	5.5
Meat, egg and fish	2.2	2.4
Vegetables and fruits	2.7	3.9
Other food	1.5	1.4
Protein intake (gms)	65	59.5

Source: Calculated from unit record data of the 38th and 55th NSSO rounds

Appendix Table A-5.1.3

Percentage Share of Food Groups in Vitamin A for Different States

State	*Cereal/ 55*	*Cereal/ 38*	*Pulses/ 55*	*Pulses/ 38*	*Mef/ 55*	*Mef/ 38*	*Vfdn/ 55*	*Vfdn/ 38*	*Milk/ 55*	*Milk/ 38*
Andhra Pradesh	2.1	10.6	2.1	3.2	5.7	2.72	66.3	53.2	14.9	17.3
Bihar	13.4	24.0	7.8	7.4	1.7	0.41	54.5	52.2	15.4	10.0
Gujarat	19.3	28.4	2.9	3.1	1.0	0.38	40.2	31.5	30.6	29.5
Haryana	6.9	14.2	2.2	2.8	0.4	0.31	34.0	26.6	44.7	41.5
Himachal Pradesh	11.0	13.7	3.8	2.9	1.2	0.51	33.9	40.4	36.6	26.9
Karnataka	8.4	15.3	2.9	3.3	3.7	1.14	58.5	52.3	18.6	14.9
Kerala	3.2	7.7	2.4	3.7	9.3	6.68	41.7	32.9	22.8	21.2
Madhya Pradesh	14.0	19.3	5.3	7.0	1.2	0.39	53.6	49.9	19.1	15.0
Maharashtra	13.8	23.5	3.9	4.9	2.9	1.50	59.7	48.6	13.9	11.0
Orissa	2.6	5.5	2.1	2.2	1.4	0.39	86.6	83.0	3.7	3.5
Punjab	4.9	7.3	2.2	2.3	1.2	0.99	38.2	35.0	32.0	31.9
Rajasthan	21.1	35.4	1.9	3.3	0.2	0.17	28.6	19.8	43.6	34.1
Tamil Nadu	2.2	15.4	2.9	3.5	6.4	2.11	61.2	54.8	13.5	10.7
Uttar Pradesh	13.8	23.0	5.0	8.8	1.5	0.42	46.1	32.7	23.0	20.4
West Bengal	2.2	4.0	3.0	2.6	7.4	1.94	78.7	83.1	6.2	5.3

Note: (55-refers to 1999-2000; 38-refers to 1983; Mef-meat, egg and fish; Vfdn-vegetables, fruits and dry fruits)

Source: Calculated from unit record data of the 38th and 55th NSSO rounds

Appendix Table A-5.1.4

Absolute Intake of Vitamin A (μg) from Food Items

Food group	*1983*	*1999-2000*
Cereal	182	122
Milk and its products	221	283
Meat, egg and fish	14	37
Vegetables and fruits	1190	1110
Other food	107	99
Total Vitamin A (μg)	1714	1651

Source: Calculated from unit record data of the 38th and 55th NSSO rounds

Appendix A-5.2

Dietary and Non-Dietary Factors Conditioning Nutritional Status

The rich individual record data of NFHS enables us to carry out the detailed analysis of nutritional status of children under three years of age and women. In this section, we give a brief account of the summary statistics of various variables—nutrient intakes and socioeconomic-environmental variables as put in Appendix Table A-5.2.1.

The detailed statistics on the type of food consumed by children under age three years reveals that almost 45 per cent of the children never consumed green leafy vegetables or fruits as complementary food which is a significant factor in determining health outcome of the child. However, 54 per cent of the children received solid or mushy food daily, and still 75 per cent of these preschool children are breastfed.

Nineteen (19) per cent of the children under age three suffered from diarrhoea and 30 per cent suffered from fever during two weeks period before the survey.

The socioeconomic status of the households to which these preschool children belong to are important factors that determine the nutritional status. A majority of the households (94%) are male-headed. Hinduism is the most popular religion with 82 per cent households as its followers, 12 per cent of the households are Muslim, and 3 per cent are Christian. 74 per cent of households belong to scheduled tribe, scheduled caste or other backward class. Mean household size of households is 7.7.

The extent of illiteracy is quite substantial as almost two-thirds of children have their mothers and one-thirds of their father as illiterate. Only 25 per cent of the fathers and 9 per cent mothers have education equal to or above high secondary class. 36 per cent of women reported having the ability to take decisions about their own health care. The employment status of mother in rural areas varies. Almost 64 per cent of the mothers are not working, 13 per cent are agricultural labourers, 15 per cent are self-employed in agriculture and rest in other allied activities. However, in contrast, more than 98 per cent of fathers are working, 49 per cent are self-employed in agriculture and 30 per cent are involved in manual activities.

In rural India, since majority of the rural households have parents living together (93%) and are male-headed (94%), one may not find their significant impact on nutritional status. Water source and sanitation have an important influence on the health of the household members, especially children. Half of the households drink water from pump, 23 per cent drink from pipe, 24 per cent drink from well and 3 per cent drink surface water. Only one-fourth of population uses some method of purifying water.

Regarding sanitation facilities, a large percentage (83%) of the households do not have any toilet facility at all. 52 per cent of the villages do not have drainage facility, while only 2 per cent of the villages have underground sewage system.

Types of house, size of the land holding and electricity connection are the indicators of standard of living, which exhibit wide variation. Only 18 per cent of the households live in *pucca* houses made up of high quality material, while 42 per cent live in *kuccha* and 40 per cent live in semi-*pucca* houses. 48 per cent of houses possess electricity connection. 35 per cent of the rural households do not own any agricultural land which is an important means of livelihood in rural areas.

Appendix Table A-5.2.1

Means and Standard Deviation of the Variables Related to Children Under Age 3 Years and their Households

Variable	*Mean*	*Standard Deviation*
Still breastfeeding	0.757	0.429
Other milk daily	0.345	0.475
Other milk some days	0.212	0.409
Other milk never	0.442	0.497
Fruit daily	0.086	0.281
Fruit some days	0.445	0.497
Fruit never	0.469	0.499
Green leafy vegetables daily	0.168	0.374
Green leafy vegetables some days	0.385	0.487
Green leafy vegetables never	0.447	0.497
Mushy food daily	0.540	0.498
Mushy food some days	0.142	0.349
Mushy food never	0.318	0.466
Single/twin	0.017	0.170
Gender (male=1)	0.520	0.500
Birth order	2.870	1.886
Age	16.936	10.224
Mother's age at birth	23.462	5.289
Had diarrhoea	0.195	0.396
Had fever	0.299	0.458
Parents living together	0.927	0.260
Woman takes health decision	0.360	0.480
BMI less than 18.5	0.429	0.495
Mother's education: Illiterate	0.630	0.483
Less than middle	0.187	0.390
Middle	0.085	0.279
Equal to high school or above	0.098	0.297
Mother's occupation if: Not working	0.639	0.480
Highly skilled jobs	0.009	0.093
Sales	0.009	0.093
Agricultural labourer	0.133	0.339
Agriculture self-employed	0.148	0.355
Physical skilled activities	0.033	0.177
Physical unskilled activities	0.030	0.171
Father's education	5.960	7.284

contd...

...contd...

Father's occupation: Self-employed in agriculture	0.487	0.500
Not working father	0.018	0.131
High skilled jobs	0.045	0.208
Clerk	0.019	0.136
Sales	0.079	0.270
Other services	0.030	0.169
Manual skilled	0.211	0.408
Manual unskilled	0.112	0.315
SC/ST households	0.742	0.932
Religion:		
Hindu	0.823	0.381
Muslim	0.128	0.334
Christian	0.022	0.146
Other religion	0.027	0.163
Sex of head (Male=1)	0.942	0.235
Household size	7.709	3.869
Percentage of children between:		
0 to 5 years	0.299	0.119
6 to 14 years	0.149	0.149
Percentage of females equal to or above 15 years	0.289	0.100
Percentage of males equal to or above 15 years	0.263	0.104
Size of landholding	3.318	10.634
Owns a *kutcha* house	0.426	0.494
Owns a *pucca* house	0.175	0.380
Owns a semi-*pucca* house	0.399	0.490
Has electricity	0.484	0.500
Pipe water	0.228	0.419
Pump water	0.495	0.500
Well water	0.240	0.427
Other sources water	0.037	0.189
Not purifying water	0.760	0.431
No toilet	0.831	0.374
Own toilet	0.148	0.355
Shared toilet	0.012	0.109
Public toilet	0.007	0.083
No drainage	0.520	0.500
Open drainage	0.455	0.498
Underground drainage	0.018	0.134
Health facility within village	0.561	0.496

Source: Calculated from unit record data of the NFHS-2 (1998-99)

6 Correlates of Nutrient Intakes

This chapter attempts to quantify the extent to which variation in the intakes of the nine nutrients being considered in this study is explained by income, demographic composition, socioeconomic status, education and occupational status of the household, and other conditioning variables. A detailed explanation of these variables and the justification for including them is provided earlier in Chapter 4. This chapter is based exclusively on unit record data of National Sample Survey (NSS) for 1983 and 1999-2000 for rural India.

A seemingly unrelated regression (SUR) framework is used in which demand functions for all nine nutrients are estimated simultaneously. We use non-parametric method (as set out in Chapter 4) to determine the use of a specification which includes both a linear and a quadratic (in logarithmic) income term. Most of the other variables capturing seasonality, socio-economic status, education, occupational status and so on are specified as dummy variables.

The SUR formulation is as follows:

$$\ln Y_{it} = \alpha_i + \beta_{1i} \ln X_t + \beta_{2i} (\ln X_t)^2 + \beta_{3i} Z_t + \varepsilon_{it}$$

where i =1 to 9 (calorie, protein, fat, iron, carotene, vitamin C, thiamine, riboflavin and niacin), t is for the t_{th} household, ln (Y_t) is the natural logarithm of per capita nutrient intake, ln (X_t) is the natural logarithm of monthly per capita expenditure and Z is the vector of other household characteristics that affect the nutrient intake of the household. The vector includes education, head of the household, sub-rounds, social status, occupational groups, household size and composition as set out in Table 4.2.

These are estimated for each state separately for 1983 and 1999-2000, enabling comparisons over time for nutrient-expenditure elasticities. The sample size consists of nearly 77,000 rural households in 1983 and 70,000 rural households in 1999-2000.

6.1 The Response to Income

As detailed in Chapter 2, the role of income in improving the nutrient intakes, especially for calories, has been a matter of debate. The evidence presented in Chapter 5 suggests that nutrient intake patterns vary substantially by quartile. Therefore, the response of nutrient intakes to income is evaluated not just at the mean but also for each quartile expenditure group. The need for this disaggregation is further reinforced by the significance of the quadratic income term for most nutrients and states (Appendix Tables A-6.1.1 and A-6.1.2). For energy, consistent with work of Meenakshi and Vishwanathan (2001), the value of the estimated parameter of the quadratic income term is found to be inevitably negative and significant for all the states. Therefore, these elasticities decline with income, a reflection of substantial curvature to the estimated Engel function.

Tables 6.1 through 6.9 present the estimated expenditure elasticities of nutrient demand, disaggregated by state and quartile and for two periods. This is for the first time such elasticities have been estimated for nutrients other than calories and proteins for India.

These nutrient-expenditure elasticities are calculated for each state at its mean and quartile incomes for 1999-2000. To make the comparison between 1983 and 1999-2000 elasticity values, we use the poverty price deflator and estimate the value of mean and quartile incomes for 1999-2000 in terms of 1983 prices. At these expenditure values, we calculate the nutrient-expenditure elasticity for 1983 and compare it with 1999-2000 values.

6.1.1 Calories

On an average, elasticities for almost all the states lie between 0.4 and 0.5 in 1999-2000. The elasticities among the poorest quartile are of the order of 0.69 and 0.64 in the poorer states of Bihar and West Bengal respectively, and are between 0.43 and 0.41 for the richest quartile as observed in Table 6.1. In other states, elasticities among the richest quartile are far lower and mostly range between 0.35 and 0.45.

Elasticities have declined on an average over time in most states except Andhra Pradesh, Maharashtra and Rajasthan where it has increased marginally. For the poorest quartile, it has not reduced for eight states and the number falls to three as one moves to higher quartile. Although decline is much less for the richer states like Punjab and Haryana than the poorer states like Bihar and Orissa.

These elasticities are comparable in magnitude to those found in the literature by Pitt (1983), Strauss (1984), Subramanian and Deaton (1996), Roy (2001) and Meenakshi and Vishwanathan (2001).

Table 6.1

Calorie Expenditure Elasticity, by State and Quartile, 1983 and 1999-2000

	*1983 (38th Round)**					*1999-2000 (55th Round)*				
State	*Q1*	*Q2*	*Q3*	*Q4*	*All*	*Q1*	*Q2*	*Q3*	*Q4*	*All*
Andhra Pradesh	0.52	0.46	0.43	0.36	0.44	0.61	0.53	0.47	0.35	0.49
Bihar	0.69	0.62	0.57	0.48	0.59	0.69	0.61	0.54	0.43	0.57
Gujarat	0.65	0.52	0.43	0.28	0.47	0.56	0.48	0.43	0.33	0.45
Haryana	0.52	0.51	0.50	0.49	0.51	0.56	0.53	0.51	0.47	0.52
Himachal Pradesh	0.58	0.50	0.44	0.33	0.47	0.36	0.36	0.36	0.36	0.36
Karnataka	0.66	0.58	0.52	0.41	0.54	0.66	0.57	0.51	0.39	0.53
Kerala	0.59	0.53	0.48	0.38	0.49	0.60	0.51	0.44	0.31	0.47
Madhya Pradesh	0.54	0.52	0.50	0.47	0.51	0.55	0.50	0.47	0.41	0.48
Maharashtra	0.43	0.40	0.37	0.32	0.38	0.54	0.46	0.39	0.28	0.42
Orissa	0.70	0.60	0.53	0.41	0.56	0.59	0.51	0.45	0.34	0.47
Punjab	0.75	0.63	0.55	0.40	0.58	0.62	0.55	0.49	0.39	0.51
Rajasthan	0.52	0.48	0.45	0.40	0.46	0.53	0.52	0.52	0.51	0.52
Tamil Nadu	0.61	0.53	0.47	0.37	0.50	0.55	0.47	0.42	0.31	0.44
Uttar Pradesh	0.58	0.54	0.51	0.46	0.52	0.56	0.50	0.46	0.38	0.47
West Bengal	0.71	0.61	0.54	0.42	0.57	0.64	0.56	0.51	0.41	0.53

Note: * Evaluated at quartile and mean incomes of 1999-2000 at 1983 prices. Q1, Q2, Q3 and Q4 refer to poorest, second, third and top quartile respectively.

6.1.2 Protein

The pattern of protein elasticities follows largely that for calories as evident in Table 6.2. For most of the states on an average, it ranges between 0.4 and 0.5 in 1999-2000. The values are much higher for the first quartile averaging around 0.5 and 0.6 than in higher quartiles where elasticities range between 0.35 and 0.45. These are comparable to the magnitudes found by Pitt (1983) for rural Bangladesh, Ward and Sanders (1980) for Northern Brazil and Meenakshi and Vishwanathan (2001).

Out of 15 states, both on an average and quartile levels, elasticities have decreased for 6 states and increased for others. In case of Andhra Pradesh, Maharashtra and Rajasthan, elasticities have increased the most, that is, by 0.1 to 0.2 points for most of the quartiles. Thus, controlling for income, the demand for proteins appears slightly more responsive to changes in income in 1999-2000 than in 1983.

Table 6.2

Protein Expenditure Elasticity, by State and Quartile, 1983 and 1999-2000

	*1983 (38th Round)**					*1999-2000 (55th Round)*				
State	*Q1*	*Q2*	*Q3*	*Q4*	*All*	*Q1*	*Q2*	*Q3*	*Q4*	*All*
Andhra Pradesh	0.55	0.49	0.46	0.39	0.47	0.64	0.56	0.51	0.41	0.53
Bihar	0.65	0.59	0.54	0.46	0.56	0.74	0.65	0.58	0.46	0.61
Gujarat	0.65	0.50	0.41	0.24	0.45	0.52	0.44	0.40	0.31	0.42
Haryana	0.55	0.50	0.47	0.41	0.48	0.54	0.51	0.48	0.44	0.49
Himachal Pradesh	0.55	0.47	0.40	0.27	0.42	0.35	0.35	0.35	0.34	0.35
Karnataka	0.63	0.56	0.51	0.41	0.53	0.64	0.56	0.50	0.38	0.52
Kerala	0.63	0.58	0.54	0.47	0.55	0.73	0.63	0.54	0.40	0.58
Madhya Pradesh	0.50	0.49	0.49	0.48	0.49	0.63	0.56	0.52	0.43	0.54
Maharashtra	0.41	0.39	0.37	0.33	0.37	0.65	0.52	0.43	0.27	0.47
Orissa	0.72	0.63	0.56	0.45	0.59	0.62	0.56	0.52	0.45	0.54
Punjab	0.75	0.62	0.51	0.34	0.56	0.58	0.52	0.47	0.39	0.49
Rajasthan	0.49	0.44	0.40	0.34	0.42	0.55	0.53	0.52	0.50	0.53
Tamil Nadu	0.61	0.53	0.47	0.37	0.50	0.64	0.55	0.48	0.36	0.51
Uttar Pradesh	0.58	0.53	0.50	0.44	0.51	0.58	0.51	0.46	0.36	0.48
West Bengal	0.66	0.58	0.54	0.45	0.56	0.72	0.64	0.58	0.48	0.61

Note: * Evaluated at quartile and mean incomes of 1999-2000 at 1983 prices. Q1, Q2, Q3 and Q4 refer to poorest, second, third and top quartile respectively.

6.1.3 Fat

The magnitudes of expenditure elasticities for fat in rural India are of much higher order as compared to calories and protein, averaging around 0.8-0.9 in 1999-2000. This high order of magnitude has also been evident in the work of Bouis and Novenario-Reese (1997) for Bangladesh. The significant negative quadratic income term in the estimated fat Engel function imparts substantial curvature to elasticities and therefore, the elasticities are higher for the poorest quartile approaching unity in many states and range between 0.8 and 0.9 as put in Table 6.3.

These elasticities have increased over time in several states except Kerala, Punjab and Orissa. Even among the poorest quartile, an increase in income elasticity can be discerned in all states except Kerala, Punjab and Orissa.

Table 6.3

Fat Expenditure Elasticity, by State and Quartile, 1983 and 1999-2000

State	*1983 (38th Round)**					*1999-2000 (55th Round)*				
	Q1	*Q2*	*Q3*	*Q4*	*All*	*Q1*	*Q2*	*Q3*	*Q4*	*All*
Andhra Pradesh	0.85	0.77	0.72	0.62	0.74	0.90	0.82	0.77	0.66	0.79
Bihar	0.71	0.74	0.76	0.80	0.75	1.04	1.01	0.98	0.94	0.99
Gujarat	0.92	0.72	0.59	0.37	0.65	0.98	0.81	0.70	0.51	0.75
Haryana	0.89	0.80	0.74	0.64	0.77	0.95	0.84	0.76	0.63	0.79
Himachal Pradesh	0.79	0.70	0.63	0.50	0.65	0.78	0.73	0.69	0.62	0.71
Karnataka	0.78	0.73	0.70	0.64	0.71	0.82	0.74	0.68	0.57	0.70
Kerala	0.97	0.88	0.80	0.67	0.83	0.90	0.78	0.68	0.50	0.72
Madhya Pradesh	0.68	0.77	0.84	0.95	0.81	1.01	0.98	0.96	0.92	0.97
Maharashtra	0.68	0.66	0.64	0.61	0.65	0.95	0.84	0.75	0.60	0.79
Orissa	1.02	0.99	0.97	0.94	0.98	0.84	0.86	0.88	0.90	0.87
Punjab	1.05	0.89	0.76	0.55	0.81	0.90	0.79	0.70	0.55	0.73
Rajasthan	0.80	0.75	0.72	0.66	0.73	0.96	0.91	0.87	0.81	0.89
Tamil Nadu	0.82	0.76	0.72	0.65	0.74	0.89	0.78	0.69	0.53	0.72
Uttar Pradesh	0.91	0.92	0.92	0.92	0.92	1.06	0.97	0.90	0.78	0.93
West Bengal	0.92	0.87	0.85	0.80	0.86	1.01	0.92	0.86	0.75	0.89

Note: * Evaluated at quartile and mean incomes of 1999-2000 at 1983 prices. Q1, Q2, Q3 and Q4 refer to poorest, second, third and top quartile respectively.

6.1.4 Iron

Observing Table 6.1 and Table 6.4, we find that expenditure elasticities of iron demand are of comparable orders of magnitude with the calorie elasticities in 1999-2000. This is hardly surprising, as cereals are the principal source for both calorie and iron intakes as discussed in section 5.2. In general, elasticities are higher among the Bihar, Madhya Pradesh, Rajasthan and Uttar Pradesh (BIMARU) states.

Between 1983 and 1999-2000, the income elasticity of iron demand has declined or stayed the same on an average in majority of the states. The exceptions are the states of Andhra Pradesh, Bihar, Gujarat, Madhya Pradesh, Maharashtra, Tamil Nadu and West Bengal, two of which are

BIMARU states. However, for the first quartile, elasticities have increased for Andhra Pradesh, Bihar, Kerala, Madhya Pradesh, Maharashtra, Orissa, Tamil Nadu and West Bengal.

Table 6.4

Iron Expenditure Elasticity, by State and Quartile, 1983 and 1999-2000

	*1983 (38th Round)**					*1999-2000 (55th Round)*				
State	*Q1*	*Q2*	*Q3*	*Q4*	*All*	*Q1*	*Q2*	*Q3*	*Q4*	*All*
Andhra Pradesh	0.39	0.36	0.34	0.30	0.35	0.51	0.44	0.39	0.30	0.41
Bihar	0.58	0.54	0.50	0.44	0.52	0.76	0.64	0.55	0.39	0.58
Gujarat	0.62	0.46	0.35	0.16	0.40	0.61	0.47	0.38	0.22	0.42
Haryana	0.41	0.39	0.37	0.33	0.37	0.38	0.34	0.31	0.27	0.32
Himachal Pradesh	0.50	0.43	0.38	0.29	0.40	0.23	0.24	0.24	0.25	0.24
Karnataka	0.60	0.53	0.47	0.38	0.50	0.58	0.51	0.46	0.36	0.48
Kerala	0.58	0.52	0.46	0.37	0.48	0.61	0.52	0.44	0.31	0.47
Madhya Pradesh	0.46	0.45	0.44	0.43	0.45	0.61	0.53	0.47	0.36	0.49
Maharashtra	0.37	0.33	0.29	0.24	0.31	0.51	0.41	0.34	0.21	0.37
Orissa	0.62	0.55	0.50	0.41	0.52	0.63	0.50	0.40	0.23	0.44
Punjab	0.67	0.54	0.44	0.28	0.48	0.48	0.43	0.38	0.31	0.40
Rajasthan	0.60	0.52	0.47	0.37	0.49	0.54	0.50	0.46	0.41	0.48
Tamil Nadu	0.47	0.40	0.35	0.25	0.37	0.50	0.42	0.37	0.27	0.39
Uttar Pradesh	0.49	0.45	0.42	0.36	0.43	0.45	0.39	0.34	0.26	0.36
West Bengal	0.59	0.53	0.49	0.42	0.50	0.65	0.57	0.52	0.43	0.54

Note: * Evaluated at quartile and mean incomes of 1999-2000 at 1983 prices. Q1, Q2, Q3 and Q4 refer to poorest, second, third and top quartile respectively.

6.1.5 Vitamin C

On an average, the expenditure elasticities of vitamin C demand are substantially higher than calorie elasticities but are lower than unity. Bouis and Novenario-Reese (1997) also obtained high expenditure elasticity of vitamin C in Bangladesh. Given that much of vitamin C is sourced primarily in fruits and vegetables, this result is somewhat surprising, as one might expect these magnitudes to exceed unity.

The quadratic income term is significantly negative in all states in 1999-2000. However, in 1983, there are few exceptions like Bihar, Orissa, Himachal Pradesh and Maharashtra which have positive quadratic income term, though it is significant only in case of Bihar (Appendix Tables A-6.1.1 and A-6.1.2).

Over time vitamin C elasticities have increased in almost all states except Haryana and Uttar Pradesh. The increase in elasticity is substantial for the poorest quartile of the BIMARU states except Uttar Pradesh which experienced a decline. In case of Bihar and Madhya Pradesh, the elasticities have increased by 0.42 points.

Table 6.5

Vitamin C Expenditure Elasticity, by State and Quartile, 1983 and 1999-2000

	*1983 (38th Round)**					*1999-2000 (55th Round)*				
State	*Q1*	*Q2*	*Q3*	*Q4*	*All*	*Q1*	*Q2*	*Q3*	*Q4*	*All*
Andhra Pradesh	0.56	0.52	0.49	0.44	0.50	0.68	0.61	0.56	0.46	0.58
Bihar	0.40	0.48	0.55	0.65	0.52	0.82	0.74	0.69	0.59	0.71
Gujarat	0.81	0.62	0.50	0.29	0.56	0.84	0.70	0.61	0.45	0.65
Haryana	0.76	0.79	0.80	0.83	0.80	1.02	0.84	0.70	0.48	0.76
Himachal Pradesh	0.41	0.42	0.42	0.44	0.42	0.83	0.73	0.65	0.51	0.68
Karnataka	0.69	0.66	0.63	0.58	0.64	0.84	0.70	0.59	0.40	0.63
Kerala	0.96	0.83	0.72	0.53	0.76	1.06	0.89	0.75	0.51	0.81
Madhya Pradesh	0.50	0.53	0.55	0.59	0.54	0.96	0.85	0.76	0.62	0.80
Maharashtra	0.71	0.61	0.53	0.39	0.56	0.85	0.74	0.65	0.51	0.69
Orissa	0.70	0.62	0.56	0.46	0.59	0.95	0.86	0.79	0.68	0.82
Punjab	0.83	0.71	0.62	0.46	0.66	0.96	0.83	0.72	0.54	0.76
Rajasthan	0.76	0.75	0.74	0.73	0.75	0.99	0.89	0.83	0.72	0.86
Tamil Nadu	0.70	0.66	0.64	0.59	0.65	0.93	0.76	0.62	0.38	0.67
Uttar Pradesh	0.98	0.88	0.81	0.68	0.84	0.79	0.73	0.69	0.62	0.71
West Bengal	0.65	0.63	0.62	0.60	0.63	0.75	0.65	0.59	0.48	0.62

Note: * Evaluated at quartile and mean incomes of 1999-2000 at 1983 prices. Q1, Q2, Q3 and Q4 refer to poorest, second, third and top quartile respectively.

6.1.6 Vitamin A (Carotene)

On an average, carotene expenditure elasticity lies between 0.65 and 0.75 for most of the states in 1999-2000. The quadratic income term is significantly negative in most of the states. Bihar, Himachal Pradesh and Orissa are exceptions in 1999-2000, which have positive quadratic term but it is not significant in any of these states. Similarly, in 1983, few states have positive income quadratic term but it is significant in case of Bihar only (Appendix Tables A-6.1.1 and A-6.1.2).

In general, the carotene expenditure elasticity declines with income and ranges between 0.5 and 0.9 for the richest quartile as observed in Table 6.6.

Besides vitamin C and fat, it is the only other nutrient whose elasticity has increased over time in majority of the states except Kerala and Gujarat. The increase is observed for almost all income groups of all states. The increase in elasticity is particularly dramatic for the first quartile of the BIMARU states. Thus, the income elasticity of vitamin A demand among the poorest 25 per cent in Bihar increased from 0.18 to 0.73.

Table 6.6

Vitamin A Expenditure Elasticity, by State and Quartile, 1983 and 1999-2000

	1983 (38th Round)*					1999-2000 (55th Round)				
State	*Q1*	*Q2*	*Q3*	*Q4*	*All*	*Q1*	*Q2*	*Q3*	*Q4*	*All*
Andhra Pradesh	0.58	0.53	0.49	0.41	0.50	0.72	0.66	0.62	0.53	0.63
Bihar	0.18	0.35	0.48	0.71	0.43	0.73	0.80	0.85	0.95	0.83
Gujarat	0.88	0.73	0.64	0.48	0.68	0.60	0.58	0.58	0.56	0.58
Haryana	0.72	0.70	0.68	0.65	0.69	1.13	0.96	0.83	0.63	0.89
Himachal Pradesh	0.19	0.25	0.30	0.38	0.28	0.56	0.58	0.59	0.61	0.59
Karnataka	0.62	0.59	0.56	0.51	0.57	1.01	0.82	0.68	0.42	0.73
Kerala	1.46	1.30	1.16	0.92	1.21	1.30	1.15	1.01	0.78	1.06
Madhya Pradesh	0.37	0.43	0.48	0.56	0.46	0.88	0.83	0.80	0.74	0.81
Maharashtra	0.52	0.50	0.48	0.45	0.49	0.76	0.67	0.60	0.48	0.63
Orissa	0.29	0.33	0.37	0.43	0.35	0.60	0.61	0.62	0.64	0.62
Punjab	0.97	0.81	0.68	0.47	0.73	0.92	0.79	0.7	0.53	0.73
Rajasthan	0.71	0.71	0.71	0.71	0.71	1.17	1.09	1.03	0.94	1.06
Tamil Nadu	0.54	0.54	0.54	0.54	0.54	1.22	0.99	0.82	0.51	0.89
Uttar Pradesh	1.06	1.03	1.01	0.96	1.01	1.23	1.14	1.07	0.94	1.10
West Bengal	0.45	0.39	0.36	0.29	0.37	0.70	0.56	0.47	0.30	0.51

Note: * Evaluated at quartile and mean incomes of 1999-2000 at 1983 prices. Q1, Q2, Q3 and Q4 refer to poorest, second, third and top quartile respectively.

6.1.7 Thiamine

Like the calorie expenditure elasticity, the average thiamine income elasticity for most of the states lies between 0.4 and 0.5 in 1999-2000. The value of the estimated parameter of the quadratic income term is found to be significantly negative for all states. Income elasticity of thiamine demand ranges between 0.4 and 0.6 for the poorest quartile and are between 0.2 and 0.3 for the richest quartile as evident in Table 6.7.

These elasticities have decreased over time in several states. Andhra Pradesh, Bihar, Madhya Pradesh, Maharashtra, Rajasthan, Tamil Nadu and West Bengal are the exceptions, three of these are BIMARU states.

Table 6.7

Thiamine Expenditure Elasticity, by State and Quartile, 1983 and 1999-2000

	*1983 (38th Round)**					*1999-2000 (55th Round)*				
State	*Q1*	*Q2*	*Q3*	*Q4*	*All*	*Q1*	*Q2*	*Q3*	*Q4*	*All*
Andhra Pradesh	0.33	0.33	0.33	0.33	0.33	0.52	0.45	0.41	0.33	0.43
Bihar	0.57	0.51	0.46	0.38	0.48	0.72	0.60	0.52	0.36	0.55
Gujarat	0.62	0.48	0.39	0.23	0.43	0.42	0.36	0.33	0.26	0.34
Haryana	0.47	0.43	0.40	0.36	0.42	0.39	0.36	0.35	0.32	0.35
Himachal Pradesh	0.55	0.44	0.36	0.20	0.39	0.25	0.24	0.24	0.23	0.24
Karnataka	0.57	0.49	0.43	0.33	0.46	0.48	0.40	0.35	0.25	0.37
Kerala	0.61	0.54	0.48	0.38	0.50	0.67	0.56	0.48	0.32	0.51
Madhya Pradesh	0.42	0.44	0.45	0.47	0.45	0.64	0.57	0.52	0.44	0.54
Maharashtra	0.33	0.31	0.28	0.25	0.29	0.55	0.43	0.35	0.20	0.38
Orissa	0.64	0.56	0.50	0.40	0.52	0.55	0.51	0.48	0.43	0.49
Punjab	0.68	0.56	0.46	0.31	0.50	0.46	0.41	0.37	0.30	0.39
Rajasthan	0.45	0.38	0.34	0.26	0.36	0.44	0.42	0.41	0.39	0.42
Tamil Nadu	0.46	0.39	0.34	0.25	0.36	0.50	0.43	0.38	0.29	0.40
Uttar Pradesh	0.48	0.44	0.41	0.35	0.42	0.47	0.40	0.35	0.26	0.37
West Bengal	0.59	0.52	0.47	0.38	0.49	0.66	0.56	0.50	0.40	0.53

Note: * Evaluated at quartile and mean incomes of 1999-2000 at 1983 prices. Q1, Q2, Q3 and Q4 refer to poorest, second, third and top quartile respectively.

6.1.8 Riboflavin

The expenditure elasticities for riboflavin, as put in Table 6.8, are slightly higher than calorie elasticities ranging between 0.5 and 0.6. The quadratic income term is negative, resulting in decline in elasticity with income. In comparison to 1983, these elasticities have declined substantially for Orissa and West Bengal, while increased in case of Andhra Pradesh, Haryana, Kerala, Madhya Pradesh, Maharashtra and Rajasthan. The states of Bihar, Gujarat, Himachal Pradesh, Punjab, Tamil Nadu and Uttar Pradesh experience marginal changes of the order of 0.01 to 0.03.

As far as poorest 25 per cent of the population is concerned, only Gujarat, Himachal Pradesh, Orissa, Punjab and West Bengal are the states that experience a decline in the elasticity, while other states experience an increase in its magnitude over time.

Table 6.8

Riboflavin Expenditure Elasticity, by State and Quartile, 1983 and 1999-2000

	*1983 (38th Round)**					*1999-2000 (55th Round)*				
State	*Q1*	*Q2*	*Q3*	*Q4*	*All*	*Q1*	*Q2*	*Q3*	*Q4*	*All*
Andhra Pradesh	0.45	0.43	0.41	0.39	0.42	0.64	0.56	0.52	0.42	0.53
Bihar	0.71	0.66	0.61	0.54	0.63	0.75	0.67	0.62	0.52	0.64
Gujarat	0.72	0.54	0.42	0.22	0.47	0.65	0.54	0.47	0.35	0.50
Haryana	0.56	0.53	0.51	0.47	0.52	0.70	0.64	0.60	0.53	0.62
Himachal Pradesh	0.57	0.51	0.45	0.36	0.47	0.47	0.46	0.45	0.44	0.45
Karnataka	0.69	0.60	0.54	0.43	0.57	0.72	0.62	0.54	0.41	0.57
Kerala	0.68	0.59	0.51	0.38	0.54	0.77	0.66	0.57	0.42	0.61
Madhya Pradesh	0.60	0.56	0.53	0.47	0.54	0.69	0.62	0.57	0.49	0.59
Maharashtra	0.49	0.44	0.40	0.33	0.41	0.59	0.51	0.44	0.33	0.47
Orissa	0.60	0.56	0.52	0.46	0.54	0.52	0.48	0.45	0.40	0.47
Punjab	0.82	0.68	0.56	0.37	0.61	0.73	0.65	0.58	0.48	0.61
Rajasthan	0.59	0.53	0.48	0.41	0.50	0.78	0.73	0.70	0.64	0.71
Tamil Nadu	0.59	0.52	0.46	0.36	0.48	0.64	0.54	0.47	0.35	0.50
Uttar Pradesh	0.64	0.59	0.55	0.48	0.56	0.66	0.60	0.55	0.46	0.57
West Bengal	0.72	0.63	0.58	0.48	0.60	0.63	0.55	0.50	0.41	0.52

Note: * Evaluated at quartile and mean incomes of 1999-2000 at 1983 prices. Q1, Q2, Q3 and Q4 refer to poorest, second, third and top quartile respectively.

6.1.9 Niacin

In the case of this nutrient as well, expenditure elasticities of niacin demand range between 0.3 and 0.4 in 1999-2000. The quadratic income term is significant and negative, imparting substantial curvature to the estimated Engel function. The elasticities among the poorest quartile are of the order of 0.67 and 0.63, and between 0.27 and 0.23 for the richest quartile in the poorer states of Bihar and Orissa respectively.

In reference to 1983, these elasticities have declined in almost all states except Maharashtra and Rajasthan, which have experienced marginal improvement of 0.03-0.04 points as observed in Table 6.9.

The poorest quartile in the poorer states of Bihar, Madhya Pradesh, Orissa, Uttar Pradesh and West Bengal have a fall in the expenditure elasticity between 0.07 and 0.10, while richer states of Gujarat, Haryana, Punjab, etc., have greater fall of 0.20 points.

Table 6.9

Niacin Expenditure Elasticity, by State and Quartile, 1983 and 1999-2000

	*1983 (38th Round)**					*1999-2000 (55th Round)*				
State	*Q1*	*Q2*	*Q3*	*Q4*	*All*	*Q1*	*Q2*	*Q3*	*Q4*	*All*
Andhra Pradesh	0.49	0.44	0.40	0.33	0.42	0.56	0.45	0.38	0.24	0.41
Bihar	0.76	0.65	0.56	0.42	0.60	0.67	0.54	0.44	0.27	0.48
Gujarat	0.76	0.59	0.48	0.30	0.53	0.56	0.46	0.40	0.29	0.43
Haryana	0.59	0.47	0.38	0.24	0.42	0.35	0.32	0.30	0.26	0.31
Himachal Pradesh	0.63	0.46	0.33	0.08	0.38	0.24	0.23	0.22	0.20	0.22
Karnataka	0.72	0.61	0.53	0.39	0.56	0.61	0.53	0.47	0.37	0.50
Kerala	0.53	0.45	0.40	0.29	0.42	0.50	0.42	0.35	0.22	0.37
Madhya Pradesh	0.56	0.50	0.45	0.37	0.47	0.54	0.45	0.38	0.26	0.41
Maharashtra	0.42	0.37	0.34	0.29	0.35	0.56	0.43	0.34	0.17	0.38
Orissa	0.74	0.56	0.43	0.22	0.49	0.63	0.50	0.40	0.23	0.44
Punjab	0.66	0.54	0.45	0.30	0.49	0.44	0.38	0.34	0.27	0.36
Rajasthan	0.52	0.44	0.39	0.30	0.42	0.49	0.47	0.45	0.42	0.46
Tamil Nadu	0.62	0.50	0.41	0.26	0.45	0.46	0.38	0.33	0.23	0.35
Uttar Pradesh	0.49	0.43	0.39	0.31	0.41	0.42	0.35	0.30	0.20	0.32
West Bengal	0.65	0.54	0.47	0.34	0.50	0.58	0.48	0.42	0.31	0.45

Note: * Evaluated at quartile and mean incomes of 1999-2000 at 1983 prices. Q1, Q2, Q3 and Q4 refer to poorest, second, third and top quartile respectively.

6.2 Occupational Status (Producer *versus* Non-producer Households)

The type of economic activity of the household influences food consumption pattern. As indicated in Table 6.10, in comparison to the base category of agricultural labour households, households self-employed in agriculture in most of the states have, *ceteris paribus*, higher intakes of fat and riboflavin only. That is, there is no significant difference for the self-employed in agriculture category in the intakes of calories, proteins, iron, vitamin C, thiamine, niacin and vitamin A. For few states, it is significant and positive for calories, proteins and vitamin A, and negative for niacin. This is also found in case of calories for rural Maharashtra by

Subramanian and Deaton (1996) and for calorie and protein by Meenakshi and Vishwanathan (2001). There is no clear pattern of difference, however, for the intakes of thiamine, vitamin C and iron for these households.

Table 6.10

Coefficients of Self–employed in Agriculture, by Nutrient and State, 1999-2000

State	*Calorie*	*Protein*	*Fat*	*Iron*	*Vitamin C*	*Vitamin A*	*Thiamine*	*Niacin*	*Riboflavin*
Andhra Pradesh	-0.01	0.01	0.09	-0.03	-0.03	0.05	0.01	-0.04	0.00
	(-0.98)	*(1.23)*	*(5.83)*	*(-2.49)*	*(-1.18)*	*(1.9)*	*(0.52)*	*(-3.60)*	*(0.24)*
Bihar	-0.01	-0.04	0.06	-0.05	0.07	0.23	-0.08	-0.04	0.02
	(-1.48)	*(-3.31)*	*(3.29)*	*(-4.02)*	*(2.48)*	*(4.82)*	*(-5.60)*	*(-3.29)*	*(2.29)*
Gujarat	0.01	0.01	0.05	-0.02	-0.01	0.07	-0.03	-0.05	0.03
	(0.42)	*(0.42)*	*(2.65)*	*(-0.63)*	*(-0.25)*	*(1.38)*	*(-1.56)*	*(-2.29)*	*(1.37)*
Haryana	-0.01	0.03	0.13	-0.03	0.01	0.03	0.00	-0.05	0.11
	(-0.33)	*(1.05)*	*(3.27)*	*(-0.93)*	*(0.15)*	*(0.32)*	*(0.15)*	*(-1.59)*	*(2.51)*
Himachal Pradesh	0.08	0.07	0.23	0.01	-0.01	0.36	0.04	0.00	0.12
	(3.33)	*(2.24)*	*(6.27)*	*(0.30)*	*(-0.08)*	*(4.98)*	*(1.33)*	*(0.06)*	*(3.18)*
Karnataka	0.05	0.05	0.11	0.04	0.01	0.13	0.07	0.04	0.07
	(3.10)	*(3.14)*	*(4.55)*	*(2.39)*	*(0.32)*	*(3.15)*	*(3.31)*	*(1.78)*	*(3.96)*
Kerala	0.02	0.02	0.14	0.00	-0.01	0.13	-0.01	0.00	0.00
	(0.95)	*(1.41)*	*(6.30)*	*(0.16)*	*(-0.25)*	*(2.23)*	*(-0.52)*	*(-0.08)*	*(0.00)*
Madhya Pradesh	0.03	0.05	0.11	0.01	-0.04	-0.06	0.06	0.02	0.04
	(3.07)	*(4.17)*	*(5.40)*	*(0.72)*	*(-1.39)*	*(-1.19)*	*(3.15)*	*(1.05)*	*(3.72)*
Maharashtra	0.01	-0.01	0.07	-0.02	-0.05	-0.07	-0.02	-0.02	0.04
	(0.48)	*(-0.80)*	*(3.01)*	*(-1.09)*	*(-1.77)*	*(-1.64)*	*(-1.24)*	*(-1.13)*	*(2.38)*
Orissa	-0.01	0.01	0.15	0.01	0.01	0.12	0.01	-0.04	0.02
	(-0.64)	*(1.21)*	*(6.53)*	*(0.50)*	*(0.14)*	*(2.01)*	*(0.61)*	*(-2.55)*	*(1.60)*
Punjab	0.02	0.04	0.08	0.00	0.05	0.02	0.02	-0.01	0.09
	(1.07)	*(1.85)*	*(2.12)*	*(0.04)*	*(1.10)*	*(0.36)*	*(1.12)*	*(-0.30)*	*(3.04)*
Rajasthan	0.00	0.02	0.08	-0.05	-0.05	0.01	-0.02	-0.07	0.03
	(0.08)	*(0.90)*	*(2.71)*	*(-1.13)*	*(-1.04)*	*(0.18)*	*(-0.74)*	*(-2.03)*	*(0.74)*
Tamil Nadu	0.05	0.05	0.11	0.02	0.03	0.12	0.06	0.01	0.08
	(3.35)	*(3.46)*	*(5.42)*	*(1.23)*	*(0.91)*	*(2.80)*	*(3.15)*	*(0.41)*	*(6.01)*
Uttar Pradesh	0.03	0.02	0.11	0.00	0.06	0.1	0.02	0.00	0.03
	(2.43)	*(1.97)*	*(6.86)*	*(0.33)*	*(2.75)*	*(3.03)*	*(1.22)*	*(-0.36)*	*(2.51)*
West Bengal	0.00	0.00	0.12	-0.01	0.02	0.06	-0.03	-0.02	0.01
	(0.00)	*(0.00)*	*(4.15)*	*(-0.63)*	*(0.34)*	*(0.77)*	*(-2.03)*	*(-1.42)*	*(0.63)*

Note: Figures in the italics refer to the value of t–ratio

Furthermore, as indicated in Appendix Tables A-6.2.1–A-6.2.3, non-producer households that are self-employed in non-agriculture, other labour and 'others" households have lower intakes of calories, protein, thiamine, niacin, riboflavin and iron in a majority of the states. Interestingly, there are no significant differences in intakes of vitamin C, vitamin A and fat for these occupational categories in reference to agricultural labour households.

In rural India, Bajpai, Sachs and Volavka (2005) have also found that people living in households cultivating 1.5 ha or more of land had calorie deficiency rates that were two-third lower than those who lived in households without land in 1999-2000.

The producer households have higher intakes of calories, protein and vitamin A, probably on account of self-consumption. Also, these households are usually involved in activities requiring more physical work and hence need more energy as compared to other households.

6.3 Seasonality

Although there is seasonality in production, there is likely to be some consumption smoothing through the year. This is easier to effect for cereals which are semi-perishable in nature than for vegetables and fruits. As cereals contribute to more than three-fourths of the calorie, protein, thiamine, niacin and iron intakes, there is likely to be less seasonal fluctuations in these nutrients as compared to vitamin C and vitamin A, which are sourced primarily in perishable vegetables and fruits.

The distribution of average nutrient intakes across seasons presented in Table 6.11 is not indicative of significant seasonality in nutrient intakes, with the exception of vitamin A and vitamin C.

Table 6.11

Level of Intakes of the Major Nutrients across Seasons, 1999-2000

Nutrient	*Average Intakes of Nutrient (per capita per day)*			
	July-September	*October-December*	*January-March*	*April-June*
Calorie (kcal)	2152	2155	2144	2128
Protein (g)	60.3	60	59.9	58.6
Fat (g)	36.2	35.8	37.0	35.7
Iron (mg)	22.2	22.5	22.4	22.4
Vitamin A (μg)	1526	1626	1854	1599
Vitamin C (mg)	51.4	66	75.9	50.1
Thiamine (mg)	1.82	1.79	1.78	1.79
Niacin (mg)	19.4	19.3	19.0	19.1
Riboflavin (mg)	1.14	1.16	1.16	1.12

Source: Calculated from unit record data of 55th NSSO rounds.

The average intakes of vitamin C are higher by almost 26 mg per capita per day in the months of January-March as compared to the summer months of April-June. Similarly, for vitamin A, average intakes are highest during January-March, with intakes higher by more than 325 μg as compared to July-September.

This pattern is confirmed at the state level as well. Table 6.12 presents the coefficients associated with seasonal dummies for vitamin A and C intakes.

Table 6.12

Coefficients of Seasonal Dummies for Iron, Vitamin A and Vitamin C Intakes, by State, 1999-2000

State	Iron			Vitamin A			Vitamin C		
	October-December	January-March	April-June	October-December	January-March	April-June	October-December	January-March	April-June
Andhra Pradesh	-0.02	-0.02	-0.01	-0.03	0.06	0.13	-0.04	-0.04	-0.13
	(-0.79)	*(-0.76)*	*(-0.32)*	*(-0.53)*	*(1.00)*	*(2.51)*	*(-0.83)*	*(-1.00)*	*(-2.93)*
Bihar	-0.02	0.01	0.02	0.20	0.41	0.33	0.20	0.63	0.10
	(-1.13)	*(0.68)*	*(0.91)*	*(2.25)*	*(4.61)*	*(3.71)*	*(3.83)*	*(14.39)*	*(2.61)*
Gujarat	0.09	0.11	0.03	-0.03	0.15	0.14	0.20	0.32	0.06
	(-1.40)	*(1.47)*	*(0.47)*	*(-0.32)*	*(2.03)*	*(1.69)*	*(2.13)*	*(3.29)*	*(0.82)*
Haryana	0.07	0.08	0.03	0.15	0.49	-0.11	0.22	0.27	-0.04
	(1.70)	*(1.47)*	*(0.81)*	*(1.49)*	*(4.93)*	*(-1.11)*	*(2.14)*	*(2.63)*	*(-0.44)*
Himachal Pradesh	-0.06	-0.07	-0.06	0.08	0.29	-0.21	0.29	0.41	0.04
	(-1.39)	*(-1.80)*	*(-1.50)*	*(0.77)*	*(2.77)*	*(-1.89)*	*(3.24)*	*(4.92)*	*(0.39)*
Karnataka	-0.04	0.00	-0.01	-0.07	0.07	0.07	-0.11	-0.09	-0.17
	(-0.75)	*(0.09)*	*(-0.16)*	*(-0.72)*	*(0.74)*	*(0.75)*	*(-1.81)*	*(-1.39)*	*(-2.54)*
Kerala	-0.02	-0.02	-0.05	0.04	-0.08	0.02	0.04	0.01	-0.03
	(-1.00)	*(-0.83)*	*(-1.97)*	*(0.68)*	*(-1.35)*	*(0.25)*	*(0.74)*	*(0.18)*	*(-0.53)*
Madhya Pradesh	-0.02	0.00	0.00	-0.09	0.26	-0.09	0.30	0.81	0.18
	(-0.80)	*(0.09)*	*(0.15)*	*(-0.96)*	*(2.88)*	*(-1.03)*	*(4.27)*	*(13.28)*	*(3.07)*
Maharashtra	0.07	0.00	-0.02	0.09	0.08	0.11	0.16	0.06	-0.10
	(1.96)	*(0.0)*	*(-0.83)*	*(1.03)*	*(1.04)*	*(1.63)*	*(2.84)*	*(1.12)*	*(-2.02)*
Orissa	0.02	0.01	0.05	0.01	-0.14	0.23	0.10	0.55	0.16
	(1.34)	*(0.29)*	*(2.39)*	*(0.10)*	*(-1.22)*	*(2.16)*	*(1.71)*	*(7.97)*	*(2.51)*
Punjab	0.07	0.11	-0.02	0.53	0.74	0.14	0.54	0.68	0.23
	(2.14)	*(3.39)*	*(-0.57)*	*(5.98)*	*(10.44)*	*(2.19)*	*(6.31)*	*(9.09)*	*(3.07)*
Rajasthan	0.03	0.01	0.05	0.28	0.45	0.15	0.26	0.37	0.05
	(0.53)	*(0.22)*	*(1.18)*	*(4.63)*	*(7.58)*	*(2.80)*	*(4.23)*	*(6.32)*	*(0.79)*
Tamil Nadu	-0.03	0.00	-0.01	-0.20	0.00	-0.05	-0.14	0.01	-0.00
	(-1.09)	*(-0.08)*	*(-0.23)*	*(-2.69)*	*(-0.06)*	*(-0.62)*	*(-2.79)*	*(0.31)*	*(-0.41)*
Uttar Pradesh	-0.01	0.05	0.04	0.03	0.55	0.07	0.34	0.84	0.25
	(-0.48)	*(2.66)*	*(2.12)*	*(0.51)*	*(8.41)*	*(1.05)*	*(7.35)*	*(21.23)*	*(6.66)*
West Bengal	0.04	0.02	0.01	0.22	0.08	0.09	0.37	0.61	0.09
	(1.63)	*(0.74)*	*(0.58)*	*(2.16)*	*(0.95)*	*(0.91)*	*(5.25)*	*(8.42)*	*(1.43)*

Note: Figures in the italics refer to the value of t–ratio

The positive coefficients associated with seasonal dummies suggest that intakes of these two micronutrients are consistently higher in January-March than in the base quarter of July-September. The supply of fresh fruits and vegetables, especially cauliflower, cabbage, carrot and green leafy vegetables, which are rich in vitamin A and vitamin C is the greatest in the winter season. Surprisingly, although mangoes, which are rich in vitamin A, are plentiful only in the summer, vitamin A intakes are not as high in these months.

For the other nutrients (see Appendix Tables A-6.3.1–A-6.3.2), there are relatively few significant coefficients. Thus, for nutrients that are sourced primarily in cereals, seasonality appears not to be significant. Seasonality in the intake of vitamin A, vitamin C and iron has also been documented by Bouis and Novenario-Reese (1997) for rural Bangladesh.

6.4 Household Size and Composition

The coefficient of the log of household size is typically negative but sometimes insignificant (Table 6.13). This negative coefficient is consistent with the results of Subramanian and Deaton (1996) for calories. The principal exception to this pattern is found in Bihar, where the coefficient is positive and significant for most nutrients. Therefore, controlling for household composition and other socioeconomic factors, larger households have lower per capita intakes of nutrient.

As far as household composition variables are concerned for nutrients sourced in cereals, a higher proportion of children in the household—male or female—is associated, as expected with lower per capita intakes in most states. This is true for all the B-vitamins (see results for thiamine in Table 6.14 and the others in Appendix Tables A-6.4.1 and A-6.4.2) as well as iron.

However, for vitamins A and vitamin C, intakes are not affected by the proportion of male and female children in the household; the associated coefficients are insignificant (see Table 6.14 and Appendix Table A-6.4.2). For macronutrients (Appendix table A-6.4.1) again , calories and proteins which are derived primarily from cereals, households with a higher proportion of children have, *ceteris paribus*, lower intakes. In the case of fats, these differences are insignificant.

The coefficient of the proportion of adult women in the household is insignificant for most nutrients and states (Appendix Tables A-4.1 and A-4.2). The important exception is iron, where the coefficient is negative and significant. This is of particular concern because iron requirements for women are higher; thus, households with more women should ideally have greater iron intakes.

Table 6.13

Coefficients of Logarithm of Household Size in Nutrient Intakes, by State, 1999-2000

State	*Calorie*	*Protein*	*Fat*	*Thiamine*	*Riboflavin*	*Niacin*	*Iron*	*Vitamin A*	*Vitamin C*
Andhra Pradesh	-0.05	-0.03	-0.11	-0.03	-0.08	-0.03	-0.09	-0.23	-0.20
	(-4.14)	*(-2.12)*	*(-6.19)*	*(-1.80)*	*(-5.14)*	*(-1.78)*	*(-4.64)*	*(-6.88)*	*(-7.59)*
Bihar	0.02	0.05	-0.01	0.06	0.04	0.04	0.04	-0.09	-0.14
	(2.48)	*(4.60)*	*(-0.39)*	*(5.03)*	*(3.02)*	*(3.80)*	*(2.94)*	*(-2.09)*	*(-4.81)*
Gujarat	-0.05	-0.05	0.01	-0.04	-0.05	-0.06	-0.04	-0.07	-0.16
	(-2.79)	*(-2.22)*	*(0.54)*	*(-1.73)*	*(-2.11)*	*(-3.15)*	*(-1.07)*	*(-1.81)*	*(-3.96)*
Haryana	-0.01	-0.01	-0.11	0.01	-0.03	0.02	0.01	-0.16	-0.13
	(-0.73)	*(-0.39)*	*(-3.10)*	*(0.35)*	*(-0.81)*	*(1.00)*	*(0.40)*	*(-2.82)*	*(-2.42)*
Himachal Pradesh	-0.05	-0.04	-0.09	-0.01	-0.07	-0.03	-0.04	-0.20	-0.17
	(-2.60)	*(-2.24)*	*(-3.79)*	*(-0.57)*	*(-3.59)*	*(-1.11)*	*(-1.96)*	*(-3.97)*	*(-3.45)*
Karnataka	-0.02	0.01	-0.03	-0.01	-0.06	0.02	-0.04	-0.18	-0.19
	(-1.10)	*(0.55)*	*(-1.31)*	*(-0.35)*	*(-3.64)*	*(0.70)*	*(-2.12)*	*(-4.18)*	*(-6.60)*
Kerala	-0.09	-0.08	-0.13	-0.10	-0.10	-0.08	-0.14	-0.09	-0.25
	(-7.03)	*(-5.11)*	*(-7.38)*	*(-6.35)*	*(-5.48)*	*(-5.00)*	*(-8.25)*	*(-2.15)*	*(-7.81)*
Madhya Pradesh	-0.03	0.01	0.04	0.04	-0.04	-0.05	-0.04	-0.13	-0.29
	(-2.47)	*(0.84)*	*(1.76)*	*(2.39)*	*(-3.24)*	*(-2.93)*	*(-2.44)*	*(-3.12)*	*(-9.36)*
Maharashtra	-0.04	-0.02	0.02	-0.02	-0.04	-0.06	-0.05	-0.13	-0.13
	(-2.22)	*(-0.63)*	*(0.58)*	*(-0.97)*	*(-2.05)*	*(-2.49)*	*(-1.89)*	*(-3.33)*	*(-4.25)*
Orissa	-0.03	-0.01	-0.15	-0.01	-0.06	0.00	-0.04	-0.32	-0.21
	(-2.37)	*(-0.85)*	*(-7.48)*	*(-0.76)*	*(-5.24)*	*(0.02)*	*(-2.95)*	*(-5.65)*	*(-6.32)*
Punjab	-0.01	0.00	-0.06	0.00	-0.01	-0.01	-0.02	-0.07	-0.09
	(-0.95)	*(0.10)*	*(-1.97)*	*(0.21)*	*(-0.24)*	*(-0.35)*	*(-1.35)*	*(-1.88)*	*(-2.09)*
Rajasthan	0.01	0.03	-0.05	0.04	0.05	0.06	0.07	0.01	-0.12
	(0.44)	*(1.97)*	*(-2.53)*	*(2.12)*	*(2.39)*	*(2.60)*	*(2.65)*	*(0.23)*	*(-3.28)*
Tamil Nadu	-0.10	-0.07	-0.10	-0.10	-0.09	-0.11	-0.16	-0.15	-0.26
	(-7.35)	*(-4.41)*	*(-5.03)*	*(-5.78)*	*(-5.78)*	*(-6.25)*	*(-8.18)*	*(-3.77)*	*(-8.29)*
Uttar Pradesh	0.00	0.00	-0.05	-0.01	0.00	0.01	-0.02	-0.03	-0.10
	(0.44)	*(0.41)*	*(-3.49)*	*(-0.79)*	*(0.03)*	*(0.93)*	*(-1.55)*	*(-1.18)*	*(-4.60)*
West Bengal	0.01	0.02	-0.09	0.02	-0.03	0.02	-0.01	-0.34	-0.22
	(0.49)	*(0.86)*	*(-3.93)*	*(0.95)*	*(-1.03)*	*(0.52)*	*(-0.44)*	*(-3.02)*	*(-6.54)*

Note: Figures in the italics refer to the value of t–ratio.

Table 6.14

Coefficients of Proportion of Adult Females, Male and Female Children in Iron, Vitamin A and Thiamine Intakes, by State, 1999-2000

State	Iron			Vitamin A			Thiamine		
	Adult Females	Male Children	Female Children	Adult Females	Male Children	Female Children	Adult Females	Male Children	Female Children
Andhra Pradesh	-0.097 *(-2.79)*	-0.142 *(-3.49)*	-0.155 *(-4.80)*	0.105 *(-1.17)*	-0.007 *(-0.09)*	0.009 *(-0.12)*	-0.081 *(-2.20)*	-0.184 *(-5.85)*	-0.184 *(-5.98)*
Bihar	-0.067 *(-1.72)*	-0.16 *(-5.26)*	-0.175 *(-5.49)*	0.132 *(0.77)*	0.01 *(0.08)*	0.197 *(1.56)*	-0.055 *(-1.45)*	-0.158 *(-5.30)*	-0.175 *(-5.50)*
Gujarat	-0.34 *(-3.12)*	-0.291 *(-3.39)*	-0.26 *(-3.08)*	-0.122 *(-0.69)*	-0.128 *(-1.19)*	-0.158 *(-1.35)*	-0.107 *(-1.64)*	-0.238 *(-4.97)*	-0.196 *(-3.94)*
Haryana	-0.286 *(-2.65)*	-0.282 *(-3.55)*	-0.249 *(-3.79)*	0.157 *(0.7)*	-0.135 *(-1.10)*	0.289 *(-1.74)*	-0.28 *(-2.82)*	-0.276 *(-3.91)*	-0.196 *(-2.97)*
Himachal Pradesh	-0.106 *(-2.25)*	-0.222 *(-5.12)*	-0.131 *(-2.77)*	0.171 *(1.32)*	-0.051 *(-0.47)*	0.134 *(1.00)*	0.03 *(-0.65)*	-0.201 *(-4.91)*	-0.069 *(-1.50)*
Karnataka	-0.081 *(-1.09)*	-0.14 *(-2.28)*	-0.105 *(-1.74)*	0.121 *(0.81)*	-0.077 *(-0.63)*	0.314 *(2.52)*	-0.139 *(-1.70)*	-0.239 *(-3.77)*	-0.181 *(-2.84)*
Kerala	-0.09 *(-2.29)*	-0.098 *(-2.33)*	-0.134 *(-2.77)*	-0.086 *(-0.74)*	0.356 *(3.13)*	0.405 *(3.50)*	-0.048 *(-1.18)*	-0.095 *(-2.32)*	-0.137 *(-2.74)*
Madhya Pradesh	-0.10 *(-2.05)*	-0.187 *(-4.86)*	-0.129 *(-3.10)*	-0.128 *(-0.84)*	-0.123 *(-1.13)*	-0.053 *(-0.46)*	-0.215 *(-3.86)*	-0.213 *(-4.59)*	-0.189 *(-3.88)*
Maharashtra	-0.039 *(-0.59)*	-0.032 *(-0.72)*	-0.157 *(-2.68)*	-0.115 *(-1.01)*	-0.10 *(-0.94)*	-0.219 *(-2.29)*	-0.034 *(-0.49)*	-0.075 *(-1.85)*	-0.196 *(-3.47)*
Orissa	-0.084 *(-2.25)*	-0.135 *(-3.44)*	-0.179 *(-4.89)*	0.412 *(2.5)*	0.251 *(1.56)*	0.474 *(2.38)*	-0.073 *(-2.13)*	-0.162 *(-5.69)*	-0.173 *(-5.13)*
Punjab	-0.094 *(-1.66)*	-0.195 *(-4.46)*	-0.156 *(-2.99)*	0.00 *(0.00)*	-0.08 *(-0.75)*	-0.244 *(-2.41)*	-0.095 *(-1.73)*	-0.172 *(-4.56)*	-0.159 *(-3.27)*
Rajasthan	-0.204 *(-2.59)*	-0.14 *(-2.58)*	-0.173 *(-2.82)*	0.045 *(0.44)*	0.136 *(1.54)*	0.009 *(0.11)*	-0.039 *(-0.62)*	-0.16 *(-3.96)*	-0.162 *(-3.51)*
Tamil Nadu	-0.014 *(-0.28)*	-0.152 *(-3.61)*	-0.195 *(-4.71)*	0.105 *(1.18)*	0.181 *(1.98)*	0.163 *(1.61)*	0.008 *(0.18)*	-0.153 *(-3.57)*	-0.224 *(-5.62)*
Uttar Pradesh	-0.144 *(-3.88)*	-0.191 *(-6.16)*	-0.236 *(-6.89)*	0.118 *(1.25)*	0.107 *(1.46)*	0.118 *(1.38)*	-0.129 *(-3.45)*	-0.201 *(-6.77)*	-0.227 *(-7.15)*
West Bengal	-0.001 *(-0.01)*	-0.075 *(-1.39)*	-0.169 *(-3.47)*	0.049 *(0.34)*	0.107 *(0.71)*	-0.14 *(-0.76)*	0.018 *(0.26)*	-0.042 *(-0.54)*	-0.147 *(-3.00)*

Note: Figures in the italics refer to the value of t–ratio

6.5 Intakes among Scheduled Caste (SC) and Scheduled Tribe (ST) Households

The literature suggests that because of social discrimination, SC and ST households have higher probability of being poor than households from other communities (Meenakshi *et al.*, 2000). If we simply compare the average intakes among SC and ST households and other households in rural

India, we find in Table 6.15 that this extends to nutrient intakes as well. On an average, SC and ST households have lower nutrient intakes than non-SC and ST households.

Table 6.15

Average Intake of Nutrients (Per Capita Per day) among SC/ST Households and Other Households in 1999-2000

Nutrient	*SC/ST Household*	*Other Household*
Calorie (kcal)	2025	2199
Protein (g)	55.9	61.1
Fat (g)	29.1	38.6
Iron (mg)	21.4	22.8
Vitamin A (μg)	1548	1695
Vitamin C (mg)	57.9	61.8
Thiamine (mg)	1.71	1.83
Niacin (mg)	18.6	19.4
Riboflavin (mg)	1.05	1.18

Source: Calculated from unit record data of 55th NSSO round.

As indicated in Table 6.16, the coefficient of the dummy variable, which takes value 1 if the household is either an SC or ST, is insignificant for most nutrients. The important exception to this is fat, where the coefficient is negative and significant in most of the states.

The coefficients of other macronutrients (calories and protein) and micronutrients (iron, vitamin C, thiamine, niacin and riboflavin) intakes are not statistically significant in most of the states. If anything, in some of the states, the coefficients for calories, protein, thiamine, niacin and iron are positive and significant. This was also the case with calories and protein in the study by Meenakshi and Vishwanathan (2001) for rural India. In contrast, the coefficients of riboflavin and vitamin A intakes, wherever significant, are often negative.

Table 6.16

Coefficients of Dummy Variable Associated with SC/ST Households in Nutrient Intakes, 1999-2000

State	Calorie	Protein	Fat	Thiamine	Riboflavin	Niacin	Iron	Vitamin A	Vitamin C
Andhra Pradesh	0.03	0.03	-0.08	0.04	0.01	0.05	0.04	-0.02	-0.03
	(3.04)	*(2.45)*	*(-5.46)*	*(3.00)*	*(0.74)*	*(4.54)*	*(3.25)*	*(-0.62)*	*(-1.20)*
Bihar	0.00	-0.03	-0.08	-0.05	0.01	0.01	0.00	0.09	-0.02
	(0.36)	*(-2.60)*	*(-4.32)*	*(-4.06)*	*(0.51)*	*(0.76)*	*(-0.20)*	*(1.69)*	*(-0.51)*
Gujarat	0.02	0.02	-0.12	-0.01	-0.15	0.07	-0.09	-0.15	-0.10
	(1.36)	*(0.65)*	*(-5.87)*	*(-0.25)*	*(-4.58)*	*(2.69)*	*(-2.04)*	*(-2.68)*	*(-1.57)*
Haryana	0.01	-0.01	-0.04	0.02	-0.04	0.03	0.04	0.03	0.01
	(0.36)	*(-0.32)*	*(-1.28)*	*(0.59)*	*(-1.02)*	*(0.94)*	*(1.19)*	*(0.52)*	*(0.09)*
Himachal Pradesh	0.02	0.02	-0.01	0.02	0.00	0.02	0.01	0.02	-0.02
	(0.86)	*(1.07)*	*(-0.43)*	*(0.80)*	*(0.18)*	*(0.89)*	*(0.29)*	*(0.37)*	*(-0.42)*
Karnataka	-0.05	-0.03	-0.05	-0.03	-0.02	-0.08	-0.04	0.02	0.03
	(-2.92)	*(-1.58)*	*(-1.87)*	*(-1.14)*	*(-1.04)*	*(-3.07)*	*(-1.57)*	*(0.41)*	*(0.73)*
Kerala	0.02	0.00	-0.07	0.03	0.02	0.03	0.01	-0.02	0.06
	(1.30)	*(0.03)*	*(-2.78)*	*(1.72)*	*(0.88)*	*(1.49)*	*(0.70)*	*(-0.30)*	*(1.44)*
Madhya Pradesh	0.00	0.00	-0.07	-0.02	-0.02	-0.01	-0.01	-0.09	0.01
	(0.15)	*(0.21)*	*(-3.07)*	*(-1.07)*	*(-1.69)*	*(-0.87)*	*(-0.84)*	*(-1.82)*	*(0.44)*
Maharashtra	0.00	0.01	-0.07	0.00	0.00	0.01	0.00	-0.10	-0.02
	(0.21)	*(0.55)*	*(-3.47)*	*(0.02)*	*(0.05)*	*(0.67)*	*(0.22)*	*(-2.40)*	*(-0.51)*
Orissa	0.02	0.02	-0.10	0.02	0.04	0.03	0.02	0.13	0.01
	(2.03)	*(2.14)*	*(-5.02)*	*(2.22)*	*(3.83)*	*(2.69)*	*(2.06)*	*(1.91)*	*(0.33)*
Punjab	0.00	0.01	-0.06	0.03	-0.02	0.03	0.03	-0.13	-0.01
	(0.11)	*(0.39)*	*(-2.01)*	*(1.49)*	*(-1.09)*	*(1.60)*	*(1.39)*	*(-2.91)*	*(-0.35)*
Rajasthan	0.01	0.01	-0.08	0.03	-0.07	-0.01	-0.04	-0.08	-0.05
	(1.11)	*(0.80)*	*(-3.68)*	*(1.88)*	*(-2.96)*	*(-0.48)*	*(-1.38)*	*(-2.16)*	*(-1.34)*
Tamil Nadu	-0.01	0.01	-0.07	0.00	-0.03	0.02	-0.01	-0.03	-0.06
	(-0.73)	*(0.47)*	*(-3.32)*	*(0.31)*	*(-2.08)*	*(1.45)*	*(-0.53)*	*(-0.71)*	*(-2.11)*
Uttar Pradesh	0.00	0.01	-0.08	0.03	-0.02	0.02	0.02	-0.10	-0.03
	(0.51)	*(0.86)*	*(-5.47)*	*(2.25)*	*(-1.78)*	*(2.03)*	*(2.00)*	*(-2.69)*	*(-1.06)*
West Bengal	0.03	0.02	-0.03	0.03	0.02	0.03	0.03	-0.01	0.02
	(2.68)	*(1.52)*	*(-1.42)*	*(2.27)*	*(1.29)*	*(2.65)*	*(1.95)*	*(-0.21)*	*(0.44)*

Note: Figures in the italics refer to the value of t–ratio

6.6 The Role of Literacy

Somewhat surprisingly, the coefficient of dummy variable representing literate household[1] is negative in the case of calories, protein, thiamine, riboflavin, niacin and iron for majority of the states[2] (Table 6.17).

1. Dummy variable takes a value 1 if any adult member of the household is literate and 0 otherwise.
2. This exercise was also tried for a different education variable, which takes value 1 if any adult member of the household has primary or above primary class education and 0 otherwise. But the sign of the dummy associated with education still appeared to be negative in most of the cases.

While apparently unexpected, the result is in line with Ravallion (1990) and Bouis and Novenario-Reese (1997), who also find negative coefficient and explain it by lower energy requirements for jobs performed by educated people contrary to positive findings of Behrman and Wolfe (1984). In our case, we control for occupational status and therefore, this explanation is not complete.

Table 6.17

Coefficients of Dummy Variable Associated with Literate Household in Nutrient Intakes, 1999-2000

State	*Calorie*	*Protein*	*Fat*	*Thiamine*	*Riboflavin*	*Niacin*	*Iron*	*Vitamin A*	*Vitamin C*
Andhra Pradesh	-0.03	-0.04	0.05	-0.06	-0.02	-0.06	-0.06	0.03	-0.01
	(-3.40)	*(-3.74)*	*(3.82)*	*(-4.79)*	*(-1.95)*	*(-5.38)*	*(-5.32)*	*(1.15)*	*(-0.45)*
Bihar	-0.02	-0.03	0.06	-0.03	-0.02	-0.04	-0.05	0.03	-0.01
	(-2.44)	*(-2.87)*	*(4.01)*	*(-3.08)*	*(-1.91)*	*(-4.18)*	*(-4.97)*	*(0.68)*	*(-0.23)*
Gujarat	-0.05	-0.06	-0.05	-0.05	-0.06	-0.03	-0.14	0.05	0.07
	(-3.01)	*(-2.66)*	*(-2.49)*	*(-2.29)*	*(-2.31)*	*(-1.16)*	*(-3.81)*	*(1.01)*	*(1.39)*
Haryana	-0.00	0.01	0.03	0.00	0.04	-0.01	-0.01	0.12	0.03
	(-0.17)	*(0.44)*	*(0.76)*	*(0.13)*	*(1.09)*	*(-0.38)*	*(-0.30)*	*(1.87)*	*(0.84)*
Himachal Pradesh	-0.02	-0.04	-0.02	-0.04	-0.05	-0.04	-0.02	0.06	0.12
	(-0.77)	*(-1.15)*	*(-0.31)*	*(-1.24)*	*(-0.89)*	*(-1.46)*	*(-0.81)*	*(0.96)*	*(1.97)*
Karnataka	-0.05	-0.07	-0.04	-0.09	-0.03	-0.08	-0.08	-0.13	0.03
	(-3.56)	*(-4.04)*	*(-1.57)*	*(-4.05)*	*(-1.58)*	*(-3.36)*	*(-3.24)*	*(-1.99)*	*(0.72)*
Kerala	0.07	0.05	0.13	0.05	0.08	0.06	0.07	-0.07	0.12
	(1.77)	*(1.14)*	*(2.68)*	*(1.10)*	*(1.85)*	*(1.46)*	*(1.70)*	*(-0.56)*	*(1.30)*
Madhya Pradesh	-0.03	-0.08	-0.09	-0.11	-0.02	0.01	-0.04	0.04	0.06
	(-3.45)	*(-7.27)*	*(-4.72)*	*(-7.38)*	*(-1.82)*	*(0.38)*	*(-2.84)*	*(1.02)*	*(1.91)*
Maharashtra	-0.04	-0.05	-0.03	-0.04	-0.05	-0.01	-0.07	0.01	0.04
	(-2.85)	*(-3.06)*	*(-1.67)*	*(-2.50)*	*(-3.14)*	*(-0.73)*	*(-3.69)*	*(0.18)*	*(1.19)*
Orissa	-0.05	-0.05	0.02	-0.07	-0.07	-0.05	-0.06	-0.04	0.01
	(-5.17)	*(-5.07)*	*(1.16)*	*(-5.74)*	*(-6.22)*	*(-4.15)*	*(-4.96)*	*(-0.56)*	*(0.34)*
Punjab	-0.05	-0.06	-0.01	-0.07	-0.06	-0.06	-0.07	-0.06	0.01
	(-3.46)	*(-4.44)*	*(-0.47)*	*(-4.69)*	*(-3.26)*	*(-3.72)*	*(-3.80)*	*(-1.23)*	*(0.27)*
Rajasthan	-0.04	-0.04	-0.05	-0.03	-0.07	-0.02	-0.08	-0.04	-0.02
	(-3.87)	*(-3.41)*	*(-2.93)*	*(-2.56)*	*(-4.02)*	*(-1.26)*	*(-3.89)*	*(-1.34)*	*(-0.56)*
Tamil Nadu	0.00	0.00	0.03	-0.03	0.00	0.00	-0.01	-0.02	0.02
	(-0.25)	*(-0.28)*	*(1.58)*	*(-1.87)*	*(-0.25)*	*(-0.34)*	*(-0.33)*	*(-0.47)*	*(0.90)*
Uttar Pradesh	-0.04	-0.04	0.03	-0.04	-0.02	-0.05	-0.05	0.02	-0.01
	(-4.02)	*(-4.49)*	*(2.50)*	*(-3.65)*	*(-2.13)*	*(-4.71)*	*(-4.25)*	*(0.81)*	*(-0.39)*
West Bengal	-0.05	-0.04	-0.04	-0.03	-0.04	-0.04	-0.05	-0.08	0.01
	(-2.65)	*(-2.04)*	*(-1.35)*	*(-1.54)*	*(-2.56)*	*(-1.75)*	*(-3.02)*	*(-1.02)*	*(0.14)*

Note: Figures in the italics refer to the value of t–ratio

Dietary habits and composition are not guided by nutritional knowledge, but rather dictated by tradition as concluded by Nilanjana Roy (2001) and this seems to be more plausible explanation in case of rural India. However, while this may result in an insignificant coefficient, this cannot explain the perverse sign.

The coefficient is insignificant for most states in case of vitamins A and C. Only in Kerala does this variable have the expected positive sign for most nutrients except vitamin A[3].

This result needs further examination for which one needs to construct a variable that captures the degree of knowledge about dietary and health care information rather than mere education levels.

6.7 Head of the Household

A dummy variable capturing difference in female- and male-headed households is insignificant in most cases as in Table 6.18. It suggests that after controlling for other socioeconomic variables, no differences in nutrient intakes can be discerned among these groups as observed by Bouis and Novenario-Reese (1997). And wherever it is significant, it is usually positive, indicating lower intakes among female-headed households. It should be noted, however, that female-headed households constitute a small minority of all households (6%).

6.8 Summary of the Main Results

As evident in previous chapter, malnutrition as computed in terms of inadequate nutrient intake continues to be a widespread problem in rural India. In this part of the research work, using the rich data source of NSS for 1983 and 1999-2000, we have analysed the determinants of the nine nutrient intakes, especially the six micronutrients at the state level for rural India. Our results suggest that nutrient elasticities are positive, though typically below one. They vary significantly by income and are high for the poorest quartile. So income is a determinant of nutrient intake among the population, especially the poor who are most deprived. This is true of all macro and micronutrients.

3. For vitamin C and niacin, it is significant at 20% level of significance.

Table 6.18

Coefficients of Dummy Variable Associated with Male-Headed Household in Nutrient Intakes, 1999-2000

State	*Calorie*	*Protein*	*Fat*	*Thiamine*	*Riboflavin*	*Niacin*	*Iron*	*Vitamin A*	*Vitamin C*
Andhra Pradesh	0.02	0.02	0	0.03	0.00	0.03	0.02	-0.03	-0.05
	(1.45)	*(1.14)*	*(-0.01)*	*(1.63)*	*(0.09)*	*(1.42)*	*(0.96)*	*(-0.78)*	*(-1.36)*
Bihar	0.02	0.04	0.03	0.08	0.01	0.03	0.05	-0.06	0.02
	(1.16)	*(2.69)*	*(1.23)*	*(4.46)*	*(0.41)*	*(1.51)*	*(2.40)*	*(-0.74)*	*(0.31)*
Gujarat	0.05	0.06	0.01	0.08	0.12	0.04	0.15	0.11	0.06
	(1.73)	*(1.51)*	*(0.35)*	*(2.14)*	*(2.03)*	*(1.21)*	*(2.18)*	*(1.58)*	*(0.45)*
Haryana	0.01	0.02	-0.04	0.04	-0.01	0.05	0.05	-0.11	-0.14
	(0.48)	*(0.53)*	*(-0.89)*	*(1.19)*	*(-0.27)*	*(1.46)*	*(1.37)*	*(-1.40)*	*(-2.23)*
Himachal Pradesh	0.01	0	0.01	0.02	-0.02	0.02	0.04	0.06	0.05
	(0.63)	*(0.11)*	*(0.24)*	*(0.84)*	*(-1.13)*	*(0.75)*	*(1.89)*	*(1.09)*	*(1.15)*
Karnataka	0.05	0.04	-0.02	0.03	0.02	0.05	0.05	0.00	0.00
	(2.38)	*(1.66)*	*(-0.60)*	*(0.97)*	*(0.68)*	*(2.33)*	*(1.92)*	*(0.00)*	*(0.09)*
Kerala	0.00	-0.01	0.00	-0.01	-0.02	0.01	0.02	-0.02	-0.01
	(0.07)	*(-0.63)*	*(0.06)*	*(-0.44)*	*(-0.93)*	*(0.51)*	*(1.32)*	*(-0.42)*	*(-0.41)*
Madhya Pradesh	0.01	-0.01	0.00	-0.01	0.00	0.00	0.01	0.01	0.10
	(0.25)	*(-0.44)*	*(0.08)*	*(0.33)*	*(-.07)*	*(0.03)*	*(0.35)*	*(0.13)*	*(1.79)*
Maharashtra	0.02	0.02	0.01	0.01	0.02	0.02	0.01	-0.02	0.02
	(-1.42)	*(0.89)*	*(0.21)*	*(0.24)*	*(0.76)*	*(0.85)*	*(0.52)*	*(-0.18)*	*(-0.47)*
Orissa	0.02	0.01	-0.1	0.04	0.01	0.03	0.04	-0.04	-0.06
	(1.20)	*(0.84)*	*(-3.96)*	*(1.82)*	*(0.43)*	*(1.79)*	*(1.87)*	*(-0.42)*	*(-0.97)*
Punjab	0.02	0.01	-0.01	0.01	-0.01	0.02	0.00	0.04	0.11
	(0.78)	*(0.28)*	*(-0.24)*	*(-0.67)*	*(-0.41)*	*(0.91)*	*(0.16)*	*(0.70)*	*(2.23)*
Rajasthan	-0.01	-0.01	0.01	0.01	0.00	0.01	0.00	0.01	0.13
	(-0.40)	*(-0.49)*	*(0.23)*	*(0.38)*	*(0.06)*	*(0.21)*	*(0.07)*	*(0.12)*	*(1.99)*
Tamil Nadu	0.04	0.03	0.01	0.03	0.03	0.04	0.04	0.00	-0.01
	(2.28)	*(1.77)*	*(0.28)*	*(1.99)*	*(1.84)*	*(2.05)*	*(1.98)*	*(0.00)*	*(-0.32)*
Uttar Pradesh	0.02	0.02	-0.01	0.02	0.02	0.04	0.02	-0.02	0.01
	(1.58)	*(1.27)*	*(-0.33)*	*(1.05)*	*(0.82)*	*(2.35)*	*(0.90)*	*(-0.32)*	*(0.20)*
West Bengal	0.03	0.05	-0.06	0.07	0.04	0.05	0.05	-0.01	0.02
	(1.44)	*(1.96)*	*(-1.76)*	*(2.31)*	*(1.42)*	*(1.98)*	*(2.36)*	*(-0.10)*	*(0.45)*

Note: Figures in the italics refer to the value of t–ratio

Elasticities for vitamin A, vitamin C and fat are higher than those for calories. For thiamine, riboflavin, niacin and protein, the magnitude of the elasticities is almost same as calories.

The nutrient-expenditure elasticities have declined over time on an average; however have increased for fat, vitamin A and vitamin C—the micronutrients that are sourced in non-staple foods.

Further, over time these elasticities have decreased in almost all states except in some of the BIMARU (poor) states, apart from Andhra Pradesh and Maharashtra.

However, for poorest quartile, the increase in the nutrient expenditure elasticities is observed in many more states.

The households self-employed in agriculture or producer households have no clear advantage in the intakes of most of the nutrients except fat and riboflavin as compared to agricultural labour households, a somewhat unexpected result.

Seasonality is an issue only for vitamins A and C, where the greater availability of seasonal fruits and vegetables during the cooler months of January-March results in higher intakes in majority of the states.

The coefficient of household is negative as expected. As far as household composition in terms of proportion of children is concerned, it matters only for cereal-sourced nutrients. The proportion of adult females in the household does not affect the per capita intake of nutrients except iron, where it is negatively significant. It is of particular concern because iron requirements of women are higher than those of others.

SC or ST households, *ceteris paribus*, have lower fat intakes as compared to other households, while no significant difference emerges for calories, protein, riboflavin, thiamine, niacin, iron, vitamin A and vitamin C intakes in majority of the states.

Somewhat surprisingly, role of literacy turns out to be negative in the case of calories, protein, thiamine, riboflavin, niacin and iron, and insignificant in the cases of vitamins A and C for most states. The explanation in terms of dietary habits guided by tradition and belief does not provide an explanation for this. It needs to be explored further.

No significant difference in nutrient intakes of female-headed and male-headed households is observed. However, wherever significant, it is indicating impoverished state of female-headed households.

Clearly, the analysis brings out the fact that behaviour of micronutrients vitamin A and C, which are primarily non-cereal based nutrients, is different, and also important is iron which is cereal based.

Appendix Table A-6.1.1

Coefficients of Log of Per Capita Total Expenditure ln (X) and its Quadratic Term (ln (X))^2 in Nutrient Intakes, 1999-2000

State	Calories		Protein		Fat		Iron		Vitamin C		Vitamin A		Thiamine		Niacin		Riboflavin	
	ln (X)	(ln (X))^2	ln (X)	(ln (X))^2	ln (X)	(ln (X))^2	ln (X)	(ln (X))^2	ln (X)	(ln (X))^2	ln (X)	(ln (X))^2	ln (X)	(ln (X))^2	ln (X)	(ln (X))^2	ln (X)	(ln (X))^2
Andhra	2.06	-0.13	1.94	-0.12	2.24	-0.12	1.7	-0.11	1.88	-0.11	1.74	-0.09	1.57	-0.1	2.3	-0.16	1.84	-0.11
Pradesh	*(11.39)*	*(-8.98)*	*(10.10)*	*(-7.64)*	*(8.76)*	*(-5.91)*	*(5.59)*	*(-4.32)*	*(3.75)*	*(-2.69)*	*(3.44)*	*(-2.33)*	*(6.32)*	*(-4.82)*	*(10.26)*	*(-8.72)*	*(8.02)*	*(-5.85)*
Bihar	2.31	-0.15	2.45	-0.16	1.64	-0.05	2.97	-0.2	2.17	-0.12	-0.6	0.12	2.9	-0.2	3.09	-0.22	2.2	-0.13
	(6.69)	*(-5.20)*	*(7.14)*	*(-5.55)*	*(3.20)*	*(-1.29)*	*(7.10)*	*(-5.84)*	*(3.48)*	*(-2.44)*	*(-0.57)*	*(1.40)*	*(7.69)*	*(-6.45)*	*(7.64)*	*(-6.65)*	*(6.40)*	*(-4.68)*
Gujarat	1.79	-0.11	1.67	-0.1	3.55	-0.23	2.7	-0.18	2.95	-0.18	0.82	-0.02	1.31	-0.08	1.98	-0.12	2.24	-0.14
	(4.14)	*(-3.25)*	*(3.01)*	*(-2.36)*	*(8.06)*	*(-6.66)*	*(4.03)*	*(-3.60)*	*(3.24)*	*(-2.72)*	*(0.65)*	*(-0.20)*	*(2.10)*	*(-1.64)*	*(4.69)*	*(-3.85)*	*(3.78)*	*(-3.12)*
Haryana	1.01	-0.04	1.07	-0.04	2.65	-0.14	0.95	-0.05	3.94	-0.25	3.85	-0.23	0.77	-0.03	0.82	-0.04	1.59	-0.08
	(1.74)	*(-0.84)*	*(2.27)*	*(-1.24)*	*(4.22)*	*(-2.94)*	*(1.87)*	*(-1.23)*	*(4.58)*	*(-3.85)*	*(4.49)*	*(-3.55)*	*(1.39)*	*(-0.74)*	*(1.40)*	*(-0.87)*	*(3.81)*	*(-2.40)*
Himachal	0.35	0	0.42	-0.01	1.64	-0.07	0.07	0.01	2.63	-0.15	0.27	0.02	0.36	-0.01	0.5	-0.02	0.62	-0.01
Pradesh	*(0.59)*	*(0.02)*	*(0.67)*	*(-0.12)*	*(2.45)*	*(-1.43)*	*(0.12)*	*(0.27)*	*(3.63)*	*(-2.84)*	*(0.33)*	*(0.41)*	*(0.54)*	*(-0.19)*	*(0.67)*	*(-0.38)*	*(0.98)*	*(-0.28)*
Karnataka	2.09	-0.13	2.06	-0.13	2.14	-0.12	1.8	-0.11	3.18	-0.21	4.18	-0.28	1.75	-0.11	1.9	-0.11	2.44	-0.15
	(5.89)	*(-4.53)*	*(5.75)*	*(-4.45)*	*(4.94)*	*(-3.49)*	*(4.38)*	*(-3.35)*	*(6.12)*	*(-5.18)*	*(3.90)*	*(-3.43)*	*(3.90)*	*(-3.21)*	*(4.57)*	*(-3.50)*	*(6.76)*	*(-5.40)*
Kerala	2.05	-0.12	2.41	-0.14	2.92	-0.17	2.13	-0.13	3.77	-0.23	3.89	-0.22	2.41	-0.15	1.89	-0.12	2.54	-0.15
	(9.80)	*(-7.80)*	*(11.66)*	*(-9.23)*	*(11.99)*	*(-9.36)*	*(7.88)*	*(-6.28)*	*(9.74)*	*(-8.21)*	*(7.59)*	*(-5.90)*	*(9.71)*	*(-8.01)*	*(7.73)*	*(-6.43)*	*(10.12)*	*(-8.01)*
Madhya	1.31	-0.07	1.63	-0.09	1.47	-0.04	1.92	-0.12	2.72	-0.16	1.62	-0.07	1.67	-0.1	2.02	-0.14	1.76	-0.1
Pradesh	*(4.81)*	*(-3.09)*	*(5.90)*	*(-4.10)*	*(2.58)*	*(-0.91)*	*(3.86)*	*(-2.93)*	*(2.92)*	*(-2.11)*	*(1.91)*	*(-1.01)*	*(4.83)*	*(-3.39)*	*(3.70)*	*(-3.07)*	*(3.94)*	*(-2.64)*
Maharashtra	1.84	-0.12	2.53	-0.17	2.68	-0.15	1.99	-0.13	2.56	-0.15	2.18	-0.13	2.31	-0.16	2.49	-0.17	1.9	-0.12
	(3.93)	*(-3.16)*	*(4.37)*	*(-3.74)*	*(3.55)*	*(-2.65)*	*(3.21)*	*(-2.74)*	*(5.44)*	*(-4.18)*	*(3.14)*	*(-2.35)*	*(4.00)*	*(-3.48)*	*(4.17)*	*(-3.69)*	*(4.63)*	*(-3.62)*
Orissa	1.82	-0.12	1.46	-0.08	0.57	0.03	1.4	-0.08	2.33	-0.13	0.43	0.02	1.16	-0.06	2.62	-0.19	1.11	-0.06
	(8.55)	*(-6.55)*	*(6.46)*	*(-4.23)*	*(1.34)*	*(0.74)*	*(5.46)*	*(-3.60)*	*(3.01)*	*(-2.06)*	*(0.39)*	*(0.17)*	*(4.48)*	*(-2.70)*	*(8.87)*	*(-7.77)*	*(4.71)*	*(-2.85)*
Punjab	1.94	-0.11	1.68	-0.09	2.86	-0.16	1.47	-0.08	3.28	-0.19	3.05	-0.18	1.34	-0.07	1.36	-0.08	2.13	-0.12
	(7.68)	*(-5.93)*	*(6.03)*	*(-4.45)*	*(8.09)*	*(-6.38)*	*(5.28)*	*(-4.04)*	*(5.14)*	*(-4.23)*	*(4.14)*	*(-3.35)*	*(5.03)*	*(-3.77)*	*(5.00)*	*(-3.90)*	*(6.40)*	*(-4.74)*
Rajasthan	0.63	-0.01	0.87	-0.03	1.94	-0.08	1.41	-0.07	2.69	-0.15	2.57	-0.12	0.73	-0.02	0.92	-0.04	1.6	-0.07
	(1.93)	*(-0.33)*	*(2.51)*	*(-1.01)*	*(4.65)*	*(-2.58)*	*(2.74)*	*(-1.88)*	*(3.97)*	*(-2.75)*	*(4.10)*	*(-2.45)*	*(1.76)*	*(-0.76)*	*(1.82)*	*(-0.94)*	*(3.60)*	*(-2.01)*
Tamil Nadu	1.68	-0.1	1.94	-0.12	2.6	-0.15	1.6	-0.1	3.55	-0.24	4.61	-0.3	1.5	-0.09	1.54	-0.1	2	-0.12
	(7.86)	*(-5.74)*	*(8.99)*	*(-6.58)*	*(6.77)*	*(-4.95)*	*(7.01)*	*(-5.36)*	*(4.77)*	*(-4.04)*	*(6.22)*	*(-5.25)*	*(6.70)*	*(-4.96)*	*(6.76)*	*(-5.29)*	*(9.52)*	*(-7.06)*
Uttar Pradesh	1.5	-0.09	1.71	-0.1	2.53	-0.13	1.49	-0.09	1.68	-0.08	2.76	-0.14	1.57	-0.1	1.59	-0.1	1.7	-0.09
	(5.21)	*(-3.63)*	*(6.60)*	*(-4.86)*	*(7.47)*	*(-4.82)*	*(4.72)*	*(-3.68)*	*(3.74)*	*(-2.26)*	*(4.15)*	*(-2.66)*	*(5.49)*	*(-4.30)*	*(5.41)*	*(-4.42)*	*(6.28)*	*(-4.29)*
West Bengal	1.93	-0.12	2.11	-0.12	2.48	-0.13	1.89	-0.11	2.29	-0.14	2.91	-0.2	2.14	-0.13	2.13	-0.14	1.89	-0.11
	(12.57)	*(-9.39)*	*(10.57)*	*(-7.82)*	*(4.28)*	*(-2.75)*	*(10.47)*	*(-7.87)*	*(4.25)*	*(-3.29)*	*(1.89)*	*(-1.68)*	*(12.01)*	*(-9.72)*	*(9.17)*	*(-7.51)*	*(10.56)*	*(-7.99*

Note: Figures in the italics refer to the value of t-ratio.

Appendix Table A-6.1.2

Coefficients of Log of Per Capita Total Expenditure ln (X) and its Quadratic Term (ln (X))² in Nutrient Intakes, 1983

State	Calories		Protein		Fat		Iron		Vitamin C		Vitamin A		Thiamine		Niacin		Riboflavin	
	ln (X)	(ln (X))²	ln (X)	(ln (X))²	ln (X)	(ln (X))²	ln (X)	(ln (X))²	ln (X)	(ln (X))²	ln (X)	(ln (X))²	ln (X)	(ln (X))²	ln (X)	(ln (X))²	ln (X)	(ln (X))²
Andhra	1.18	-0.08	1.23	-0.08	1.8	-0.11	0.75	-0.04	1.32	-0.09	1.05	-0.06	0.36	0.00	1.18	-0.08	0.68	-0.03
Pradesh	*(6.48)*	*(-4.13)*	*(5.97)*	*(-3.73)*	*(7.88)*	*(-4.79)*	*(3.76)*	*(-2.09)*	*(3.98)*	*(-2.63)*	*(4.18)*	*(-2.23)*	*(2.12)*	*(-0.18)*	*(6.10)*	*(-3.97)*	*(3.85)*	*(-1.54)*
Bihar	1.68	-0.12	1.57	-0.11	0.27	0.05	1.24	-0.08	-2.32	0.3	-0.8	0.14	1.5	-0.11	2.39	-0.19	1.54	-0.1
	(12.68)	*(-8.01)*	*(11.66)*	*(-7.47)*	*(1.25)*	*(2.15)*	*(8.06)*	*(-4.68)*	*(-3.94)*	*(4.75)*	*(-2.10)*	*(3.57)*	*(9.37)*	*(-6.39)*	*(16.98)*	*(-12.28)*	*(9.38)*	*(-5.52)*
Gujarat	2.15	-0.17	2.39	-0.2	3.17	-0.26	2.54	-0.22	2.51	-0.19	2.99	-0.25	2.24	-0.19	2.68	-0.22	2.79	-0.24
	(7.45)	*(-5.85)*	*(7.13)*	*(-6.00)*	*(9.41)*	*(-7.42)*	*(8.10)*	*(-6.95)*	*(4.08)*	*(-3.07)*	*(4.84)*	*(-4.04)*	*(6.10)*	*(-5.09)*	*(6.81)*	*(-5.54)*	*(10.56)*	*(-8.82)*
Haryana	0.64	-0.01	1.1	-0.06	1.95	-0.12	0.72	-0.03	1.00	-0.03	0.46	0.03	0.95	-0.05	2.03	-0.16	0.96	-0.04
	(1.71)	*(-0.34)*	*(2.69)*	*(-1.51)*	*(3.60)*	*(-2.10)*	*(1.45)*	*(-0.70)*	*(1.52)*	*(-0.48)*	*(0.73)*	*(0.55)*	*(1.85)*	*(-1.05)*	*(1.39)*	*(-1.13)*	*(2.99)*	*(-1.34)*
Himachal	1.68	-0.12	1.77	-0.13	2.04	-0.14	1.4	-0.1	-0.65	0.09	0.27	0.01	2.1	-0.17	3.04	-0.27	1.52	-0.1
Pradesh	*(3.68)*	*(-2.70)*	*(3.80)*	*(-2.95)*	*(5.45)*	*(-3.73)*	*(3.51)*	*(-2.52)*	*(-0.86)*	*(1.28)*	*(0.43)*	*(0.24)*	*(3.43)*	*(-2.90)*	*(3.20)*	*(-2.80)*	*(3.59)*	*(-2.51)*
Karnataka	1.66	-0.12	1.55	-0.11	1.34	-0.06	1.51	-0.11	1.08	-0.05	1.18	-0.06	1.55	-0.11	2.08	-0.16	1.76	-0.12
	(7.76)	*(-5.17)*	*(7.48)*	*(-4.93)*	*(4.41)*	*(-2.02)*	*(6.86)*	*(-4.63)*	*(2.56)*	*(-1.21)*	*(3.75)*	*(-1.75)*	*(5.94)*	*(-4.26)*	*(7.10)*	*(-5.28)*	*(7.22)*	*(-4.81)*
Kerala	1.38	-0.09	1.24	-0.07	2.17	-0.13	1.4	-0.09	3.56	-0.23	2.62	-0.18	1.47	-0.09	1.42	-0.1	1.84	-0.13
	(10.12)	*(-6.18)*	*(7.03)*	*(-3.74)*	*(9.69)*	*(-5.83)*	*(9.27)*	*(-5.74)*	*(5.36)*	*(-3.56)*	*(5.43)*	*(-3.94)*	*(8.06)*	*(-5.03)*	*(7.68)*	*(-5.18)*	*(6.84)*	*(-4.64)*
Madhya	0.85	-0.05	0.71	-0.04	0.96	-0.03	0.86	-0.06	0.79	-0.03	1.93	-0.14	0.65	-0.04	0.91	-0.06	1.09	-0.07
Pradesh	*(5.22)*	*(-2.79)*	*(4.39)*	*(-2.01)*	*(4.91)*	*(-1.53)*	*(4.86)*	*(-3.05)*	*(2.34)*	*(-0.90)*	*(5.98)*	*(-4.27)*	*(3.74)*	*(-1.99)*	*(5.06)*	*(-3.01)*	*(6.81)*	*(-4.13)*
Maharashtra	0.8	-0.03	0.59	-0.01	-0.35	0.13	0.6	-0.02	-0.35	0.09	0.15	0.04	0.23	0.02	1.27	-0.09	1.12	-0.06
	(3.23)	*(-1.24)*	*(2.21)*	*(-0.38)*	*(-1.43)*	*(5.01)*	*(2.71)*	*(-0.72)*	*(-0.70)*	*(1.75)*	*(0.29)*	*(0.83)*	*(0.77)*	*(0.78)*	*(4.48)*	*(-2.92)*	*(4.80)*	*(-2.60)*
Orissa	1.83	-0.13	1.8	-0.13	1.34	-0.04	1.43	-0.1	-0.27	0.07	1.64	-0.11	1.57	-0.11	2.76	-0.24	1.14	-0.06
	(10.53)	*(-7.29)*	*(8.81)*	*(-5.86)*	*(4.45)*	*(-1.20)*	*(5.96)*	*(-3.81)*	*(-0.36)*	*(0.83)*	*(2.30)*	*(-1.49)*	*(5.87)*	*(-3.98)*	*(7.48)*	*(-5.81)*	*(3.63)*	*(-1.94)*
Punjab	2.26	-0.16	2.49	-0.19	3.21	-0.23	2.33	-0.18	3.07	-0.23	2.42	-0.17	2.22	-0.17	2.17	-0.17	2.73	-0.21
	(3.98)	*(-3.00)*	*(3.99)*	*(-3.15)*	*(4.36)*	*(-3.34)*	*(3.41)*	*(-2.75)*	*(5.92)*	*(-4.71)*	*(3.51)*	*(-2.68)*	*(3.60)*	*(-2.82)*	*(3.60)*	*(-2.82)*	*(4.75)*	*(-3.76)*
Rajasthan	1.05	-0.06	1.2	-0.08	1.48	-0.08	1.68	-0.12	0.67	0.00	0.92	-0.02	1.32	-0.1	1.54	-0.12	1.48	-0.1
	(3.56)	*(-2.01)*	*(4.72)*	*(-3.15)*	*(5.11)*	*(-2.57)*	*(5.64)*	*(-4.13)*	*(2.07)*	*(0.11)*	*(2.49)*	*(-0.50)*	*(3.84)*	*(-2.87)*	*(4.11)*	*(-3.12)*	*(8.25)*	*(-5.55)*
Tamil Nadu	1.54	-0.11	1.51	-0.1	1.45	-0.07	1.28	-0.09	0.54	0.00	1.08	-0.04	1.24	-0.09	1.97	-0.15	1.47	-0.1
	(7.74)	*(-4.88)*	*(8.80)*	*(-5.49)*	*(6.14)*	*(-2.82)*	*(6.81)*	*(-4.58)*	*(1.67)*	*(0.01)*	*(3.88)*	*(-1.53)*	*(6.57)*	*(-4.41)*	*(7.74)*	*(-5.46)*	*(8.58)*	*(-5.36)*
Uttar Pradesh	1.07	-0.06	1.16	-0.07	0.88	0.00	1.03	-0.06	1.43	-0.04	2.16	-0.14	1.02	-0.06	1.22	-0.09	1.27	-0.08
	(7.69)	*(-3.93)*	*(7.82)*	*(-4.41)*	*(6.13)*	*(0.27)*	*(7.17)*	*(-4.19)*	*(4.70)*	*(-1.43)*	*(7.54)*	*(-4.86)*	*(6.46)*	*(-3.81)*	*(7.60)*	*(-5.05)*	*(9.11)*	*(-5.13)*
West Bengal	2.01	-0.15	1.57	-0.11	1.47	-0.06	1.34	-0.09	1.16	-0.08	0.88	-0.03	1.56	-0.11	2.02	-0.16	1.79	-0.12
	(11.41)	*(-7.67)*	*(10.54)*	*(-6.23)*	*(5.56)*	*(-2.02)*	*(7.92)*	*(-4.49)*	*(0.86)*	*(-0.58)*	*(1.64)*	*(-0.44)*	*(9.42)*	*(-6.00)*	*(10.62)*	*(-7.54)*	*(7.16)*	*(-4.56)*

Note: Figures in the italics refer to the value of t–ratio

Appendix Table A-6.2.1

Coefficients of Occupational Status in Energy, Protein and Fat Intakes, 1999-2000

State	*Calories*			*Protein*			*Fat*		
	Senal	*Othlab*	*Others*	*Senal*	*Othlab*	*Others*	*Senal*	*Othlab*	*Others*
Andhra Pradesh	-0.04	-0.07	-0.09	-0.02	-0.06	-0.09	0.02	-0.03	0.04
	(-2.86)	*(-4.21)*	*(-5.25)*	*(-1.33)*	*(-3.71)*	*(-5.88)*	*(0.75)*	*(-1.63)*	*(1.87)*
Bihar	-0.04	-0.02	-0.06	-0.04	-0.06	-0.07	0.00	-0.12	0.01
	(-3.25)	*(-1.14)*	*(-3.84)*	*(-3.32)*	*(-2.69)*	*(-4.30)*	*(0.20)*	*(-2.74)*	*(0.66)*
Gujarat	-0.05	-0.03	-0.10	-0.06	-0.03	-0.14	-0.03	-0.08	-0.05
	(-2.50)	*(-0.84)*	*(-4.00)*	*(-2.53)*	*(-0.66)*	*(-4.65)*	*(-1.12)*	*(-2.93)*	*(-1.78)*
Haryana	-0.09	-0.03	-0.11	-0.10	-0.02	-0.09	0.02	-0.06	0.00
	(-3.41)	*(-0.82)*	*(-4.06)*	*(-3.05)*	*(-0.30)*	*(-2.81)*	*(0.51)*	*(-1.46)*	*(0.03)*
Himachal Pradesh	0.06	0.07	0.02	0.03	0.04	-0.02	0.22	0.18	0.17
	(1.98)	*(2.29)*	*(0.55)*	*(0.71)*	*(1.04)*	*(-0.56)*	*(4.66)*	*(3.38)*	*(4.16)*
Karnataka	-0.06	-0.11	-0.04	-0.06	-0.11	-0.06	0.04	-0.15	0.09
	(-3.02)	*(-3.30)*	*(-1.49)*	*(-2.66)*	*(-2.89)*	*(-1.89)*	*(1.42)*	*(-3.60)*	*(2.20)*
Kerala	-0.03	-0.02	-0.06	-0.01	-0.02	-0.05	0.09	0.00	0.11
	(-2.29)	*(-1.43)*	*(-4.07)*	*(-0.56)*	*(-0.95)*	*(-2.87)*	*(4.31)*	*(-0.12)*	*(4.98)*
Madhya Pradesh	-0.06	-0.06	-0.09	-0.06	-0.03	-0.07	0.06	0.00	0.01
	(-2.36)	*(-2.73)*	*(-4.90)*	*(-2.60)*	*(-0.74)*	*(-2.38)*	*(1.36)*	*(0.02)*	*(0.44)*
Maharashtra	-0.10	-0.11	-0.12	-0.12	-0.14	-0.18	-0.02	-0.07	0.00
	(-5.73)	*(-3.85)*	*(-4.56)*	*(-5.73)*	*(-4.14)*	*(-5.55)*	*(-0.85)*	*(-2.22)*	*(0.12)*
Orissa	-0.02	-0.05	-0.08	0.00	-0.05	-0.06	0.02	0.04	0.13
	(-1.59)	*(-2.11)*	*(-4.58)*	*(0.28)*	*(-2.14)*	*(-3.07)*	*(0.68)*	*(1.19)*	*(4.98)*
Punjab	-0.07	-0.04	-0.03	-0.09	-0.07	-0.06	-0.02	-0.01	0.05
	(-3.09)	*(-1.89)*	*(-1.65)*	*(-3.33)*	*(-3.46)*	*(-2.71)*	*(-0.57)*	*(-0.17)*	*(1.38)*
Rajasthan	-0.08	-0.06	-0.10	-0.08	-0.05	-0.09	-0.05	-0.08	-0.06
	(-3.46)	*(-2.48)*	*(-3.86)*	*(-3.71)*	*(-2.03)*	*(-3.22)*	*(-1.63)*	*(-2.32)*	*(-1.59)*
Tamil Nadu	-0.05	-0.04	-0.06	-0.05	-0.04	-0.05	0.04	0.05	0.13
	(-3.17)	*(-2.71)*	*(-3.66)*	*(-2.89)*	*(-2.65)*	*(-2.97)*	*(2.03)*	*(2.01)*	*(4.80)*
Uttar Pradesh	-0.06	-0.05	-0.06	-0.05	-0.03	-0.06	-0.03	0.00	0.05
	(-4.45)	*(-3.04)*	*(-3.79)*	*(-3.77)*	*(-1.88)*	*(-3.83)*	*(-1.71)*	*(-0.05)*	*(2.15)*
West Bengal	-0.04	-0.04	-0.09	-0.02	-0.03	-0.08	0.08	-0.01	0.14
	(-2.93)	*(-2.76)*	*(-4.92)*	*(-1.25)*	*(-1.77)*	*(-4.68)*	*(2.91)*	*(-0.25)*	*(3.88)*

Note: Figures in the italics refer to the value of t–ratio

Senal refers to self-employed in non-agriculture, Othlab refers to other labour, Others refer to other categories.

Appendix Table A-6.2.2

Coefficients of Occupational Status in Iron, Vitamin A and Vitamin C Intakes, 1999-2000

State	*Iron*			*Vitamin A*			*Vitamin C*		
	Senal	*Othlab*	*Others*	*Senal*	*Othlab*	*Others*	*Senal*	*Othlab*	*Others*
Andhra Pradesh	-0.03	-0.06	-0.07	0.01	0.05	-0.01	0.02	-0.01	-0.07
	(-1.67)	*(-3.05)*	*(-2.67)*	*(0.42)*	*(1.06)*	*(-0.20)*	*(0.73)*	*(-0.32)*	*(-2.23)*
Bihar	-0.07	-0.07	-0.08	0.06	-0.23	0.11	-0.05	-0.21	0.02
	(-4.68)	*(-2.85)*	*(-3.80)*	*(1.08)*	*(-1.97)*	*(1.62)*	*(-1.55)*	*(-3.75)*	*(0.5)*
Gujarat	-0.07	-0.1	-0.17	-0.03	-0.05	-0.08	-0.05	-0.09	-0.05
	(-1.76)	*(-1.95)*	*(-3.73)*	*(-0.61)*	*(-0.60)*	*(-1.16)*	*(-1.00)*	*(-0.96)*	*(-1.1)*
Haryana	-0.12	-0.05	-0.12	-0.09	-0.12	-0.17	-0.04	-0.08	-0.02
	(-2.53)	*(-0.72)*	*(-2.92)*	*(-1.16)*	*(-1.45)*	*(-1.95)*	*(-0.52)*	*(-0.93)*	*(-0.25)*
Himachal Pradesh	-0.02	0	-0.05	0.38	0.36	-0.38	0.02	-0.02	-0.08
	(-0.60)	*(-0.02)*	*(-1.19)*	*(4.29)*	*(3.95)*	*(-4.66)*	*(0.2)*	*(-0.13)*	*-0.66*
Karnataka	-0.06	-0.1	-0.05	0.1	-0.15	-0.01	-0.02	-0.28	-0.13
	(-2.56)	*(-2.16)*	*(-1.44)*	*(1.59)*	*(-1.37)*	*(-0.18)*	*(-0.47)*	*(-4.81)*	*(-2.54)*
Kerala	-0.05	0	-0.09	0.11	0.04	0.16	-0.07	-0.05	-0.1
	(-2.64)	*(-0.07)*	*(-3.96)*	*(2.25)*	*(0.71)*	*(2.89)*	*(-1.51)*	*(-1.40)*	*(-2.10)*
Madhya Pradesh	-0.07	-0.09	-0.08	-0.06	-0.04	-0.05	0.04	-0.17	-0.12
	(-2.81)	*(-2.38)*	*(-2.38)*	*(-0.78)*	*(-0.37)*	*(-0.72)*	*(0.83)*	*(-2.02)*	*(-1.97)*
Maharashtra	-0.1	-0.13	-0.13	-0.09	-0.17	-0.04	0.03	0.04	-0.01
	(-4.62)	*(-3.41)*	*(-3.67)*	*(-1.64)*	*(-2.18)*	*(-0.70)*	*(0.65)*	*(0.8)*	*(-0.19)*
Orissa	-0.01	-0.04	-0.07	-0.08	-0.04	-0.06	-0.01	0.02	0
	(-0.40)	*(-1.57)*	*(-3.37)*	*(-1.03)*	*(-0.29)*	*(-0.67)*	*(-0.15)*	*(0.31)*	*(0.04)*
Punjab	-0.09	-0.06	-0.07	-0.05	-0.05	-0.04	0.02	0.04	-0.04
	(-2.86)	*(-2.51)*	*(-2.85)*	*(-1.02)*	*(-0.76)*	*(-0.83)*	*(0.50)*	*(0.70)*	*(-0.83)*
Rajasthan	-0.11	-0.18	-0.16	-0.1	-0.19	-0.16	-0.05	-0.11	-0.05
	(-2.33)	*(-3.26)*	*(-3.02)*	*(-1.58)*	*(-2.72)*	*(-2.26)*	*(-1.07)*	*(-1.73)*	*(-0.84)*
Tamil Nadu	-0.08	-0.06	-0.11	-0.02	0.09	-0.13	-0.1	-0.02	-0.06
	(-4.57)	*(-3.16)*	*(-4.97)*	*(-0.65)*	*(1.83)*	*(-2.53)*	*(-2.88)*	*(-0.64)*	*(-1.52)*
Uttar Pradesh	-0.06	-0.01	-0.07	0	0.13	0.06	0.02	0.07	0.05
	(-3.74)	*(-0.72)*	*(-3.76)*	*(-0.02)*	*(2.19)*	*(1.11)*	*(0.59)*	*(1.70)*	*(1.29)*
West Bengal	-0.05	-0.03	-0.12	-0.02	-0.07	0	0.01	0.06	-0.07
	(-2.87)	*(-1.64)*	*(-6.20)*	*(-0.21)*	*(-0.68)*	*(0.01)*	*(0.12)*	*(0.95)*	*(-1.31)*

Note: Figures in the italics refer to the value of t–ratio

Senal refers to self-employed in non-agriculture, Othlab refers to other labour, Others refer to other categories.

Appendix Table A-6.2.3

Coefficients of Occupational Status in Thiamine, Riboflavin and Niacin Intakes, 1999-2000

State	Thiamine			Riboflavin			Niacin		
	Senal	Othlab	Others	Senal	Othlab	Others	Senal	Othlab	Others
Andhra Pradesh	-0.03	-0.05	-0.09	-0.03	-0.06	-0.07	-0.06	-0.06	-0.15
	(-1.66)	*(-2.43)*	*(-5.31)*	*(-1.99)*	*(-3.65)*	*(-3.86)*	*(-3.87)*	*(-3.18)*	*(-7.37)*
Bihar	-0.06	-0.08	-0.09	-0.03	-0.05	-0.02	-0.04	-0.02	-0.07
	(-4.37)	*(-2.67)*	*(-4.80)*	*(-2.43)*	*(-2.39)*	*(-0.76)*	*(-3.03)*	*(-0.97)*	*(-3.89)*
Gujarat	-0.07	-0.02	-0.15	-0.06	-0.1	-0.13	-0.05	-0.07	-0.12
	(-2.68)	*(-0.44)*	*(-4.81)*	*(-2.18)*	*(-2.73)*	*-3.75*	*(-2.18)*	*(-2.62)*	*-4.04*
Haryana	-0.1	-0.02	-0.09	-0.11	-0.06	-0.08	-0.11	-0.02	(-0.11)
	(-2.69)	*(-0.29)*	*-2.58*	*(-2.63)*	*(-0.84)*	*(-1.77)*	*(-2.93)*	*(-0.39)*	*-3.16*
Himachal Pradesh	0	0.04	-0.05	0.05	0.06	-0.03	-0.04	-0.02	(-0.07)
	(-0.06)	*(0.95)*	*(-1.32)*	*(-1.32)*	*(-1.35)*	*(-0.79)*	*(-1.13)*	*(-0.60)*	*-1.82*
Karnataka	-0.07	-0.14	-0.05	-0.06	-0.13	(-0.05)	-0.06	-0.12	(-0.08)
	(-2.80)	*(-2.97)*	*(-1.4)*	*(-2.70)*	*(-3.45)*	*(-1.6)*	*(-2.48)*	*(-2.56)*	*-2.2*
Kerala	-0.06	-0.03	-0.1	-0.06	-0.04	-0.08	-0.05	-0.02	-0.09
	(-3.32)	*(-1.51)*	*(-4.48)*	*(-3.06)*	*(-1.97)*	*(-3.75)*	*(-2.46)*	*(-1.05)*	*(-4.55)*
Madhya Pradesh	-0.05	-0.01	-0.05	-0.07	-0.09	-0.1	-0.08	-0.13	-0.1
	(-1.72)	*(-0.23)*	*(-0.99)*	*(-3.62)*	*(-3.34)*	*(-4.88)*	*(-3.17)*	*(-3.02)*	*(-3.73)*
Maharashtra	-0.14	-0.16	-0.19	-0.07	-0.1	-0.07	-0.1	-0.09	-0.16
	(-5.98)	*(-4.08)*	*(-5.68)*	*(-4.05)*	*(-3.44)*	*(-2.69)*	*(-4.11)*	*(-2.58)*	*(-4.93)*
Orissa	0.01	-0.04	-0.05	-0.01	-0.04	-0.05	-0.02	-0.06	-0.11
	(-0.6)	*(-1.73)*	*(-2.91)*	*(-0.86)*	*(-1.58)*	*-2.78*	*(-1.23)*	*(-2.25)*	*(-5.47)*
Punjab	-0.08	-0.08	-0.06	-0.09	-0.1	-0.05	-0.1	-0.07	-0.07
	-2.85)	*(-2.98)*	*(-2.54)*	*(-3.10)*	*(-4.16)*	*(-2.09)*	*(-3.37)*	*(-2.92)*	*(-2.98)*
Rajasthan	-0.08	-0.04	-0.12	-0.12	-0.15	-0.13	-0.08	-0.14	-0.10
	(-3.10)	*(-1.64)*	*(-4.11)*	*(-3.50)*	*(-3.53)*	*(-3.07)*	*(-2.24)*	*(-3.60)*	*(-2.84)*
Tamil Nadu	-0.06	-0.06	-0.09	-0.05	-0.03	-0.03	-0.07	-0.05	-0.12
	(-3.19)	*(-3.22)*	*(-4.59)*	*(-3.01)*	*(-1.91)*	*(-1.61)*	*(-3.81)*	*(-2.68)*	*(-5.48)*
Uttar Pradesh	-0.05	-0.02	-0.07	-0.07	-0.05	-0.03	-0.06	-0.06	-0.09
	(-3.36)	*(-0.93)*	*(-3.95)*	*(-4.67)*	*(-2.38)*	*(-1.45)*	*(-3.68)*	*(-2.92)*	*(-4.75)*
West Bengal	-0.03	-0.02	-0.11	-0.03	-0.04	-0.07	-0.05	-0.05	-0.15
	(-1.85)	*(-0.80)*	*(-5.62)*	*(-1.50)*	*(-1.85)*	*(-3.61)*	*(-3.38)*	*(-2.58)*	*(-7.16)*

Note: Figures in the italics refer to the value of t–ratio

Senal refers to self-employed in non-agriculture, Othlab refers to other labour, Others refer to other categories.

Appendix Table A-6.3.1

Coefficients of Seasonal Dummies for Energy, Protein and Fat Intakes, 1999-2000

State	Energy			Protein			Fat		
	Oct-Dec	Jan-March	Apr-June	Oct-Dec	Jan-March	Apr-June	Oct-Dec	Jan-March	Apr-June
Andhra Pradesh	-0.009	-0.016	-0.025	-0.023	-0.013	-0.034	-0.01	0	-0.02
	(-0.59)	*(-0.95)*	*(-1.61)*	*(-1.39)*	*(-0.67)*	*(-2.02)*	*(-0.64)*	*(-0.02)*	*(-0.78)*
Bihar	-0.042	-0.027	-0.019	-0.055	-0.063	-0.022	-0.05	-0.02	0.03
	(-2.62)	*(-1.71)*	*(-1.26)*	*(-2.97)*	*(-3.54)*	*(-1.18)*	*(-1.74)*	*(-0.79)*	*-1.02*
Gujarat	0.026	0.031	-0.026	0.015	0.039	-0.065	0.01	0.04	0.02
	(-0.68)	*(0.83)*	*(-0.73)*	*(0.29)*	*(0.75)*	*(-1.28)*	*(0.37)*	*(0.89)*	*(0.55)*
Haryana	0.044	0.019	0.001	0.084	0.046	0.053	0.09	0.1	-0.03
	(1.69)	*(0.54)*	*(0.03)*	*(2.41)*	*(1.03)*	*(1.7)*	*(2.28)*	*(2.79)*	*(-0.66)*
Himachal Pradesh	0.012	-0.009	-0.029	0.016	0.006	-0.03	0.05	0.03	-0.04
	(0.4)	*(-0.36)*	*(-1.09)*	*(0.44)*	*(0.19)*	*(-0.84)*	*(1.11)*	*(-0.82)*	*(-1.02)*
Karnataka	-0.026	-0.007	0.002	-0.014	-0.007	0.004	-0.01	0.01	0.03
	(-0.79)	*(-0.27)*	*(0.07)*	*(-0.38)*	*(-0.20)*	*(0.12)*	*(-0.22)*	*(0.27)*	*(0.7)*
Kerala	-0.016	-0.014	-0.034	-0.043	-0.035	-0.072	0	0.01	0.01
	(-0.84)	*(0.73)*	*(-1.88)*	*(-2.07)*	*(-1.60)*	*(-3.39)*	*(-0.07)*	*(0.22)*	*(0.43)*
Madhya Pradesh	-0.003	0.006	-0.033	-0.018	0.005	-0.03	0.04	0.01	-0.05
	(-0.15)	*(0.3)*	*(-1.75)*	*(-0.60)*	*(0.2)*	*(-1.05)*	*(0.9)*	*(0.23)*	*(-1.17)*
Maharashtra	0.015	-0.004	-0.038	0.022	-0.008	-0.047	0.02	0.01	-0.03
	(0.79)	*(-0.19)*	*(-1.96)*	*(0.88)*	*(-0.28)*	*(-1.88)*	*(0.65)*	*(0.18)*	*(-1.03)*
Orissa	0.015	0.011	0.013	0.001	0.018	0.009	-0.03	0.04	0.06
	(0.97)	*(0.7)*	*(0.82)*	*(0.08)*	*(1.12)*	*(0.55)*	*(-0.79)*	*(1.33)*	*(1.81)*
Punjab	-0.01	0.032	-0.08	0.015	0.047	-0.083	-0.02	0.07	-0.08
	-0.41)	*1.22*	*(-3.25)*	*(0.61)*	*(1.82)*	*(-3.10)*	*(-0.65)*	*(-2.01)*	*(-2.26)*
Rajasthan	0.018	0.001	0.007	0.013	-0.016	0.019	0.05	0.06	-0.04
	(0.77)	*(0.07)*	*(0.34)*	*(0.51)*	*(-0.73)*	*(0.86)*	*(1.52)*	*(1.74)*	*(-1.31)*
Tamilnadu	-0.011	-0.007	-0.021	-0.024	-0.008	-0.027	-0.05	-0.04	-0.02
	(-0.56)	*(-0.36)*	*(-1.01)*	*(-1.33)*	*(-0.43)*	*(-1.32)*	*(-1.81)*	*(-1.44)*	*(-0.94)*
Uttar Pradesh	0.016	0.055	0.01	-0.013	0.025	-0.015	0.07	0.1	0.04
	(-1.07)	*(3.64)*	*(0.69)*	*(-0.81)*	*(1.52)*	*(-0.92)*	*(3.22)*	*(4.56)*	*(2.15)*
West Bengal	0.011	0.011	0.014	0.008	0.01	-0.008	0.04	0.02	0.05
	(0.61)	*(0.59)*	*(0.72)*	*(0.39)*	*(0.55)*	*(-0.44)*	*(1.07)*	*(0.66)*	*(1.42)*

Note: Figures in the italics refer to the value of t–ratio

Senal refers to self-employed in non-agriculture, Othlab refers to other labour, Others refer to other categories.

Appendix Table A-6.3.2

Coefficients of Seasonal Dummies for Thiamine, Riboflavin and Niacin Intakes, 1999-2000

State	*Thiamine*			*Riboflavin*			*Niacin*		
	Oct-Dec	*Jan-March*	*Apr-June*	*Oct-Dec*	*Jan-March*	*Apr-June*	*Oct-Dec*	*Jan-March*	*Apr-June*
Andhra Pradesh	-0.016	-0.01	-0.016	-0.033	-0.037	-0.049	0.001	-0.034	-0.026
	(-0.78)	*(-0.43)*	*(-0.74)*	*(-1.78)*	*(-1.87)*	*(-2.75)*	*0.04*	*(-1.69)*	*(-1.30)*
Bihar	-0.059	-0.08	-0.015	-0.04	-0.007	-0.005	-0.04	-0.028	-0.021
	(-2.63)	*(-3.71)*	*(-0.70)*	*(-2.06)*	*(-0.41)*	*(-0.28)*	*(-1.98)*	*(-1.43)*	*(-1.12)*
Gujarat	0.043	0.045	-0.042	0.006	0.094	-0.03	0.027	0.008	-0.037
	(.87)	*(0.88)*	*(-0.88)*	*(0.12)*	*(1.52)*	*(-0.58)*	*(0.73)*	*(0.18)*	*(-0.94)*
Haryana	0.039	0.028	0.046	0.133	0.081	0.061	0.027	0.009	0.02
	(1.09)	*(0.62)*	*(1.39)*	*(2.84)*	*(1.51)*	*(1.41)*	*(0.7)*	*(0.18)*	*(0.64)*
Himachal Pradesh	0.007	0	-0.018	-0.048	-0.07	-0.109	-0.078	-.077	-0.045
	(0.17)	*(-0.01)*	*(-0.43)*	*(-1.27)*	*(-2.21)*	*(-3.12)*	*(1.59)*	*(-1.91)*	*(1.06)*
Karnataka	-0.005	0.011	-0.007	-0.037	-0.016	-0.02	-0.019	-0.037	0.015
	(-0.10)	*0.25*	*(-0.18)*	*(-1.07)*	*(-0.49)*	*(-0.68)*	*(-0.42)*	*(-0.85)*	*(0.36)*
Kerala	-0.021	-0.015	-0.052	-0.006	-0.023	-0.053	-0.035	-0.014	-0.05
	(-0.81)	*(-0.59)*	*(-2.16)*	*(-0.21)*	*(-0.84)*	*(-1.99)*	*(-1.65)*	*(-0.62)*	*(-2.32)*
Madhya Pradesh	-0.035	-0.006	-0.016	0.002	0.043	-0.024	-0.033	-0.012	-0.025
	(-0.84)	*(-0.14)*	*(-0.39)*	*(0.07)*	*(2.01)*	*(-1.00)*	*(-1.06)*	*(-0.46)*	*(-0.90)*
Maharashtra	0.012	-0.02	-0.033	0.056	0.009	-0.049	0.008	0.028	-0.04
	(0.39)	*(-0.59)*	*(-1.05)*	*(2.13)*	*(0.37)*	*(-2.28)*	*(0.32)*	*(0.98)*	*(-1.54)*
Orissa	0.009	0.033	0.031	0.01	0.026	0.029	0.026	0.015	-0.001
	(0.43)	*(1.65)*	*(.41)*	*(0.55)*	*(1.39)*	*(1.65)*	*(1.51)*	*(0.78)*	*(-0.03)*
Punjab	0.017	0.05	-0.068	0.056	0.074	-0.055	0.021	0.055	-0.072
	(0.61)	*(1.7)*	*(-2.49)*	*(1.89)*	*(2.55)*	*(-1.68)*	*(0.72)*	*(1.77)*	*(-2.56)*
Rajasthan	-0.024	-0.041	0.029	0.044	0.014	0.007	-0.08	-0.085	0.056
	(-0.79)	*(-1.47)*	*(1.1)*	*(1.05)*	*(0.35)*	*(0.21)*	*(-1.75)*	*(-1.89)*	*(1.43)*
Tamilnadu	-0.018	-0.012	-0.018	-0.022	-0.021	-0.022	0.002	0.007	-0.007
	(-0.76)	*(-0.48)*	*(-0.66)*	*(-1.20)*	*(-1.09)*	*(-1.05)*	*(0.1)*	*(0.27)*	*(-0.28)*
Uttar Pradesh	-0.047	-0.003	-0.017	0.03	0.083	0.011	-0.014	0.018	-0.015
	(-2.40)	*(-0.16)*	*(-0.91)*	*(1.8)*	*(4.6)*	*(0.73)*	*(-0.69)*	*(0.93)*	*(-0.76)*
West Bengal	-0.004	0.008	-0.004	0.048	0.068	0.036	0.024	0.019	0.009
	(-0.18)	*(0.39)*	*(-0.20)*	*(1.69)*	*(2.75)*	*(1.55)*	*(1.05)*	*(0.87)*	*(0.37)*

Note: Figures in the italics refer to the value of t–ratio

Senal refers to self-employed in non-agriculture, Othlab refers to other labour, Others refer to other categories.

Appendix Table A-6.4.1

Coefficients of Demographic Composition for Energy, Protein and Fat Intakes, 1999-2000

State	Energy			Protein			Fat		
	Adult Females	Male Children	Female Children	Adult Females	Male Children	Female Children	Adult Females	Male Children	Female Children
Andhra Pradesh	-0.081	-0.149	-0.147	-0.078	-0.155	-0.137	0.051	0.004	0.036
	(-2.41)	*(-5.41)*	*(-5.31)*	*(-2.16)*	*(-5.62)*	*(-4.68)*	*(1.1)*	*(0.1)*	*(.93)*
Bihar	-0.034	-0.127	-0.14	-0.031	-0.107	-0.131	0.074	0.071	0.066
	(-1.13)	*(-5.88)*	*(-5.52)*	*(-0.94)*	*(-4.27)*	*(-4.62)*	*(1.43)*	*(1.72)*	*(1.38)*
Gujarat	-0.08	-0.17	-0.185	-0.068	-0.181	-0.166	0.055	0.049	-0.02
	(-1.44)	*(-4.27)*	*(-4.70)*	*(-1.10)*	*(-3.78)*	*(-3.70)*	*(0.74)*	*(0.85)*	*(-0.37)*
Haryana	-0.204	-0.228	-0.144	-0.257	-0.247	-0.122	-0.068	-0.116	0.062
	(-2.65)	*(-4.10)*	*(-2.74)*	*(-2.75)*	*(-3.80)*	*(-1.74)*	*(-0.53)*	*(-1.26)*	*(0.68)*
Himachal Pradesh	0.047	-0.148	-0.043	0.06	-0.12	0	0.191	-0.049	0.136
	(.29)	*(-4.01)*	*(-1.06)*	*(1.28)*	*(-2.84)*	*(0.01)*	*(0.22)*	*(-0.84)*	*(2.00)*
Karnataka	-0.041	-0.127	-0.106	-0.062	-0.142	-0.106	0.102	-0.076	-0.055
	(-0.76)	*(-2.82)*	*(-2.21)*	*(-1.00)*	*(-2.66)*	*(-2.04)*	*(1.33)*	*(-1.23)*	*(-0.92)*
Kerala	-0.033	-0.106	-0.124	0.003	-0.002	0.01	0.073	0.061	0.084
	(-1.05)	*(-3.57)*	*(-2.99)*	*(0.09)*	*(-0.06)*	*(0.19)*	*(1.4)*	*(1.29)*	*(1.69)*
Madhya Pradesh	-0.031	-0.188	-0.148	-0.118	-0.2	-0.166	-0.185	-0.024	-0.109
	(-0.80)	*(-6.65)*	*(-4.79)*	*(-2.66)*	*(-5.90)*	*(-4.40)*	*(-2.45)*	*(-0.44)*	*(-1.81)*
Maharashtra	-0.014	-0.082	-0.167	-0.032	-0.056	-0.17	0.049	-0.014	-0.075
	(-0.29)	*(-2.57)*	*(-3.71)*	*(-0.49)*	*(-1.47)*	*(-3.31)*	*(0.65)*	*(-0.32)*	*(-1.26)*
Orissa	-0.074	-0.172	-0.191	-0.056	-0.135	-0.137	0.124	0.104	0.146
	(-2.59)	*(-6.70)*	*(-6.73)*	*(-1.74)*	*(-5.05)*	*(-4.59)*	*(2.16)*	*(1.8)*	*(2.48)*
Punjab	-0.106	-0.141	-0.145	-0.079	-0.134	-0.179	-0.063	-0.04	-0.104
	(-2.27)	*(-3.66)*	*(-3.75)*	*(-1.50)*	*(-3.61)*	*(-4.14)*	*(-0.73)*	*(-0.58)*	*(-1.65)*
Rajasthan	-0.03	-0.121	-0.11	-0.018	-0.138	-0.109	0.082	0.021	0.054
	(-0.66)	*(-3.91)*	*(-3.07)*	*(-0.35)*	*(-3.69)*	*(-2.62)*	*(1.41)*	*(0.41)*	*(1.04)*
Tamil Nadu	0.003	-0.157	-0.194	0.038	-0.118	-0.169	0.009	-0.008	-0.05
	(.08)	*(-4.57)*	*(-5.24)*	*(0.91)*	*(-3.31)*	*(-4.68)*	*(0.17)*	*(-0.18)*	*(-1.01)*
Uttar Pradesh	-0.048	-0.153	-0.155	-0.079	-0.153	-0.172	-0.019	-0.006	0.013
	(-1.62)	*(-6.40)*	*(-5.97)*	*(-2.40)*	*(-5.58)*	*(-6.08)*	*(-0.38)*	*(-0.16)*	*(0.3)*
West Bengal	0.005	-0.064	-0.138	-0.002	-0.016	-0.106	0.116	-0.01	-0.054
	(.08)	*(-1.11)*	*(-4.29)*	*(-0.04)*	*(-0.23)*	*(-2.61)*	*(1.98)*	*(-0.14)*	*(-0.72)*

Note: Figures in the italics refer to the value of t–ratio

Appendix Table A-6.4.2

Coefficients of Demographic Composition for Vitamin C, Niacin and Riboflavin Intakes, 1999-2000

State	Vitamin C			Niacin			Riboflavin		
	Adult Females	*Male Children*	*Female Children*	*Adult Females*	*Male Children*	*Female Children*	*Adult Females*	*Male Children*	*Female Children*
Andhra Pradesh	0.104	-0.102	-0.044	-0.095	-0.22	-0.204	-0.068	-0.127	-0.128
	(1.36)	*(-1.67)*	*(-0.82)*	*(-2.57)*	*(-7.30)*	*(-6.60)*	*(-1.92)*	*(-3.82)*	*(-4.27)*
Bihar	0.064	-0.05	-0.042	-0.054	-0.182	-0.196	-0.021	-0.111	-0.105
	(0.71)	*(-0.71)*	*(-0.56)*	*(-1.57)*	*(-6.59)*	*(-6.31)*	*(-0.56)*	*(-4.07)*	*(-3.58)*
Gujarat	0.017	-0.1	-0.027	-0.138	-0.285	-0.212	-0.158	-0.146	-0.15
	(0.17)	*(-1.17)*	*(-0.30)*	*(-2.48)*	*(-5.41)*	*(-4.32)*	*(-2.07)*	*(-2.51)*	*(-2.66)*
Haryana	0.028	0.011	0.073	-0.294	-0.288	-0.281	-0.231	-0.212	-0.051
	(0.15)	*(0.09)*	*(0.53)*	*(-2.93)*	*(-3.67)*	*(-4.14)*	*(-1.88)*	*(-2.56)*	*(-0.51)*
Himachal Pradesh	0.082	-0.121	-0.04	-0.089	-0.193	-0.097	0.074	-0.068	0.069
	(0.85)	*(-1.08)*	*(-0.33)*	*(-1.70)*	*(-3.95)*	*(-1.80)*	*(1.51)*	*(-1.55)*	*(1.2)*
Karnataka	0.322	-0.021	0.135	0.013	-0.084	-0.054	0.018	-0.093	-0.066
	(2.66)	*(-0.21)*	*(1.74)*	*(0.19)*	*(-1.37)*	*(-0.90)*	*(0.25)*	*(-1.61)*	*(-1.21)*
Kerala	-0.075	0.157	0.088	-0.042	-0.153	-0.193	-0.034	-0.049	-0.083
	(-0.81)	*(1.59)*	*(1.03)*	*(-1.05)*	*(-4.16)*	*(-3.96)*	*(-0.71)*	*(-0.92)*	*(-1.76)*
Madhya Pradesh	0.11	0.094	0.059	0.004	-0.226	-0.119	-0.025	-0.145	-0.091
	(1.04)	*(1.18)*	*(0.72)*	*(0.08)*	*(-5.71)*	*(-2.80)*	*(-0.54)*	*(-4.20)*	*(-2.37)*
Maharashtra	0.104	-0.07	-0.01	0.002	-0.076	-0.174	-0.03	-0.031	-0.16
	(1.31)	*(-1.03)*	*(-0.13)*	*(0.03)*	*(-1.95)*	*(-3.17)*	*(-0.62)*	*(-0.80)*	*(-3.25)*
Orissa	0.239	0.089	0.203	-0.068	-0.207	-0.223	-0.06	-0.148	-0.139
	(2.24)	*(1.06)*	*(2.03)*	*(-1.96)*	*(-6.11)*	*(-6.63)*	*(-1.90)*	*(-5.01)*	*(-4.15)*
Punjab	-0.002	-0.143	-0.019	-0.101	-0.174	-0.162	-0.079	-0.129	-0.193
	(-0.02)	*(-1.49)*	*(-0.22)*	*(-1.85)*	*(-4.41)*	*(-3.20)*	*(-1.17)*	*(-2.57)*	*(-3.70)*
Rajasthan	0.146	0.035	0.03	-0.102	-0.154	-0.184	-0.075	-0.074	-0.091
	(1.34)	*(0.37)*	*(0.31)*	*(-1.27)*	*(-2.74)*	*(-3.03)*	*(-1.23)*	*(-1.50)*	*(-1.65)*
Tamil Nadu	0.153	0.19	0.034	0.022	-0.208	-0.237	0.007	-0.097	-0.162
	(2.04)	*(2.79)*	*(0.44)*	*(0.5)*	*(-5.32)*	*(-5.65)*	*(0.18)*	*(-2.67)*	*(-4.35)*
Uttar Pradesh	-0.158	-0.14	-0.065	-0.093	-0.216	-0.232	-0.042	-0.092	-0.118
	(-1.93)	*(-2.28)*	*(-0.99)*	*(-2.36)*	*(-7.07)*	*(-6.81)*	*(-1.12)*	*(-2.86)*	*(-3.68)*
West Bengal	-0.033	-0.072	-0.175	0	-0.049	-0.137	-0.018	-0.069	-0.157
	(-0.34)	*(-0.68)*	*(-1.44)*	*(0)*	*(-0.59)*	*(-2.91)*	*(-0.28)*	*(-1.07)*	*(-2.90)*

Note: Figures in the italics refer to the value of t–ratio

7 Correlates of Nutritional Status

There is a growing literature which focuses attention not just on nutrient intakes but on nutritional status as well. This literature highlights the role of other determinants such as a clean living environment, health and caring practices, and dietary quality, in addition to nutrient intakes in explaining the nutritional status.

Empirical work on this question in India has been limited in large part because of the lack of systematic data on nutritional status. The principal sources of such data are the surveys conducted by the National Institute of Nutrition, but these are limited to 10 states and contain information aggregated to the state level. Another relatively underutilised source is the National Family Health Survey (NFHS) which is nationally representative, and therefore, forms the bedrock for the nutritional status and living environment indicators used in this chapter.

Here we analyse the results of two different exercises: firstly, in section 7.1, using the fixed effect model as described in section 4.4.1, we identify the determinants of nutritional status of children under the age of three years using the individual-level NFHS data; and secondly, in section 7.2, using the canonical correlation analysis, we find out the factors associated with prevalence of undernourishment among the women between 15-49 years of age and children under the age of 3 years using the regional-level data set constructed from both the NFHS and National Sample Survey (NSS) surveys.

7.1 Correlates of Nutritional Status among Children under the Age of 3 Years

The nutritional status of children below three years of age is measured by standardised weight-for-age z-score. For preschool children, the dietary intake variables considered include breastfeeding status and frequency of complementary diet—consumption of green leafy vegetables, fruits and mushy food. As noted earlier, it is not possible to derive nutrient intakes from NFHS data; these variables serve as a proxy for nutrient intake.

Among non-nutrient variables that affect the actual absorption or utilisation of nutrients, we have considered the health status of the child—whether he suffered from diarrhoea or fever in the past two weeks. The other socioeconomic variables which operate at individual, parent, household and village specific levels are age, gender, birth order, age of the mother, parental education, occupational status of the parents, power of the mother, nutritional status of the mother, whether parents are living together or not, household size and composition, size of the land holding, type of house, provision of electricity, sex of the head, religion and ethnicity of the household, source of water (pipe, pump, well, and other sources) and provision of sanitation facilities, accessibility to health facilities, and sewerage system of the village.

We use a fixed effect specification, implemented at the state, village, household and parent levels for estimation. The justification for the use of variables and methodology has been discussed in section 4.4.2. The sample size is more than 18,000 children under the age of three years living in 2,531 villages in 25 Indian states.

The results have been analysed in terms of changes in standardised weight-for-age *z*-score and also in changes in weight of the male child of age nine months whose weight is less than reference median weight. These are presented in Table 7.1.

7.1.1 The Role of Child-specific Variables

Nutrient Intakes

Table 7.1 shows that feeding practices related to breastfeeding and quality of complementary food significantly influence the nutritional status of the children in the family. Children who are breastfed have higher weight-for-age scores than children who are not being breastfed. This is consistent with other studies by Melville *et al.* (1988) and Greiner and Latham (1981) that underscore the importance of breast milk in ensuring positive nutritional outcomes for young children. Thus, a breastfed reference nine-month old boy would weigh 50 g more than reference child who is not breastfed.

Children who consume green leafy vegetables daily or sometimes have a higher weight-for-age z-score than who do not consume. Further, children who consume fruits daily have better nutritional status as compared to those who do not consume. Interestingly, there is no significant difference in the nutritional status of the children who are fed solid food (mushy food) or other milk daily or sometimes and those who are not.

According to WHO (1998), in developing countries, children aged 1-2 years obtain, on an average, more than half of their daily energy requirements from breast milk. Thus, it appears that quality of complementary foods rather than energy density matters more for ensuring better nourished children.

To put the numbers in perspective, a reference male child would improve his weight by 164 g if green leafy vegetables are consumed daily or by 155 g if given green leafy vegetables sometimes compared to reference male child who did not consume any green leafy vegetables. This suggests that in addition to the quality of the complementary food, frequency of its intake is also an important determinant of nutritional status.

Non-dietary Child-specific Variables

The age of the child and age squared are significant, implying that the child's nutritional status has U-shaped relationship with the age and the turn occurring at the age of two years and three months. This is consistent with the other studies examining the relationship between age and nutritional status. For example, Maxwell *et al.* (2000) and Yimer (2000) find that nutritional status has U-shaped relationship with age.

It is also evident from the fact that percentage of children between 6-11 months of age, who are undernourished in rural India, is 40 per cent and it increases to 61 per cent for children between 12-23 months of age (NFHS, 1998-99).

Birth order of the child turns out to be negatively associated with nutritional status of the child. This is expected—as the birth order rank increases, the child has to compete for maternal care and resources with the siblings and that adversely affects his health outcome, as is evident from the work of Horton (1988) and Wolfe and Behrman (1987).[1]

Table 7.1

Regression Estimates for Standardised Weight-for-Age Z-Score

Variables	*Coefficient*	*t-value*	*Change in terms of weight of male child whose age is 9 months and has weight less than median weight*
Child-specific Factors			
Nutrient intakes			
Still breastfeeding	0.051	2.16	0.050
Other milk daily	0.006	0.13	0.006
Other milk some days	0.013	0.26	0.013
Fruit daily	0.189	1.81	0.183
Fruit some days	0.07	0.92	0.067
Green leafy vegetables daily	0.169	1.90	0.164
Green leafy vegetables some days	0.16	2.02	0.155
Mushy food daily	0.005	0.06	0.005
Mushy food some days	-0.041	-0.47	-0.040
Non-dietary variables			
Age of child (months)	-0.215	-18.33	-0.208
Square of child's age	0.004	17.02	0.004
Birth order	-1.045	-12.46	-1.01
Gender (Male=1)	-0.007	-0.1	-0.007
Birth order * gender	0.048	2.19	0.047
Had diarrhoea	-0.069	-1.39	-0.067
Had fever	0.045	0.94	0.043
Single/Twin	-0.014	-0.15	-0.013
Parent-specific Factors			
Mother's age at birth (years)	0.337	3.26	0.325
Square of mother's age	-0.004	-2.33	-0.003
Parents living together	0.51	4.13	0.49
Woman takes health decision	0.39	3.83	0.378
BMI less than 18.5	-0.17	-2.27	-0.168
Mother's education			
Less than middle	-0.04	-0.38	-0.042
Middle	-0.52	-3.5	-0.506
Equal to high school or above	-0.45	-2.73	-0.43

contd...

1. Only 4 per cent of the households who have high standard of living have birth order of five as compared to 54 per cent of the households having low standard of living. High birth order children are disproportionately from lower socioeconomic strata which are already hard pressed for resources.

...contd...

Mother's occupation			
Highly skilled jobs	-0.21	-0.56	-0.202
Sales	1.44	1.63	1.396
Agricultural labourer	0.66	3.21	0.635
Agriculture self-employed	0.72	5.02	0.699
Physical skilled activities	1.01	3.26	0.977
Physical unskilled activities	1.26	3.37	1.219
Father's education	-0.01	-1.47	-0.01
Father's occupation			
Not working father	-0.18	-0.83	-0.173
High skilled jobs	-0.23	-1.2	-0.222
Clerk	0.42	1.73	0.403
Sales	0.053	0.32	0.05
Other services	-0.12	-0.58	-0.116
Manual skilled	-0.01	-0.05	-0.006
Manual unskilled	0.56	3.15	0.54
Household-specific Characteristics			
SC/ST	-0.063	-4.13	-0.061
Religion			
Muslim	-0.054	-0.99	-0.052
Christian	0.150	1.58	0.145
Other religion	0.200	2.44	0.193
Sex of head (Male=1)	-0.056	-1.09	-0.054
Household size	0.021	6.09	0.021
Percentage of children between 0 to 5 years	-0.004	-3.11	-0.0041
Percentage of children between 6 to 14 years	-0.0105	-8.7	-0.0101
Percentage of females equal to or above 15 years	0.0065	3.6	0.0063
Size of landholding	0.005	5.08	0.0052
Owns a *pucca* house	0.349	8.25	0.337
Owns a semi-*pucca* house	0.162	4.94	0.157
Has electricity	0.303	9.21	0.293
Pipe water	0.151	2.25	0.146
Pump water	0.073	1.06	0.070
Well water	0.054	0.79	0.053
Not purifying water	-0.126	-3.82	-0.122
Own toilet	0.490	12.23	0.473
Shared toilet	0.389	4.30	0.376
Public toilet	0.371	2.47	0.358
Village-specific Characteristics			
Open drainage	-0.041	-1.72	-0.040
Underground drainage	-0.072	-0.83	-0.070
Health facility within village	0.036	1.53	0.034

No gender bias is evident as the dummy variable for the gender of the child is not significant. However, when interaction with the birth order is allowed for, it turns out to be significantly positive, indicating bias in favour of male child. It is also found in the work of Behrman (1987, 1988). In other words, the weight-for-age z-score of the male child would be greater than female child of any birth order by 0.048 standard deviation units, or a reference male child of age of 9 months would have an advantage of 47 g of weight as compared to his female counterpart.

Ill health of a child can contribute to poor nutritional status on account of loss of appetite or greater waste (Svedberg, 2000; Martorell *et al.*, 1980 and Waterlow and Tomkins, 1992). In our study, the coefficient of dummy variable representing occurrence of diarrhoea in the past week is negative, indicating an inverse relationship between weight-for-age z-score and diarrhoea, but it is insignificant. It could be that the episodes of fever and /or diarrhoea are not severe enough to be reflected in weight loss.

7.1.2 The Role of Parent-specific Variables

Mother's age which is to serve as a proxy for experience in caring for a child turns out to be significant along with square of her age in determining the nutritional status of the child. It exhibits an inverted U-shaped relationship, indicating that very young and old mothers have less ability to meet the care for their children who thus have poorer weight-for-age scores.

Households in which couple is staying together have better nourished children as compared to households in which parents are living separately. However, nearly 93 per cent of rural children in India have parents who live together.

The empowerment of the mother in the house is found to be positively associated with the nutritional status of the child. The literature suggests that women are more likely to spend more of their income on family welfare and food (Haddad *et al.*, 1996; Thomas, 1997). Our results indicate that women who report being able to take decisions on health have children with better nutritional status.

The nutritional status of the mother is also related to that of her child (Engle *et al.*, 1999; Martorell *et al.*, 1998; WHO, 1995). The weight-for-age z-score of a child whose mother is undernourished is lower than a child whose mother is well nourished. The reference male child of well nourished mother weighs 168 g more than that of undernourished mother.

One does not find any significant difference in the nutritional status of the children whose mothers are illiterate or less than middle level educated. However, contrary to the perceived wisdom, the coefficient of middle or above middle level educated mothers turns out to be perverse. It may imply that getting education may not mean gaining nutritional knowledge and thus, improving nutritional status.

Women self-employed in agriculture or agriculture labourers or manually skilled or unskilled workers have better nourished children as compared to non-working mothers. The probable explanation could be greater accessibility to food, either on account of payment in-kind or self-consumption, which may result in better nutritional status of children.

Father's education is not found to be significant in influencing the nutritional status of the child. Similarly, there is no difference between nutritional status of the children whose fathers are involved in highly skilled jobs, sales, other services, or as clerks, manually skilled or self-employed in agriculture, except for children of manually unskilled labour. This underscores the primacy of the education and occupation of mother than father in determining the nutritional status of their children.

7.1.3 The Role of Household-specific Variables

The dummy variable for SC/ST/OBC households is negative and significant, indicating that such children weigh less than their non-SC/ST counterpart. The weight of reference male child belonging to SC/ST/OBC communities is 61 g lower than in other communities.

The estimated coefficients of dummy variables associated with different religions show that there is no difference between the nutritional status of Hindu, Christian and Muslim children, while Sikh, Jain and Buddhist children are better nourished than Hindu children. A reference male child belonging to other religions would weigh 193 g more than a Hindu male child.

The coefficient of the gender of the head is insignificant, indicating that there is no difference between the nutritional status of the children belonging to male-headed households or female-headed households. Once again, only a very small percentage of households is female-headed in the sample.

Household size is also found to be positively related to child's nutritional status in rural India. Larger households have nutritionally better off children than smaller sized households, perhaps, on account of economies of scale. This result may also be seen in the study of Behrman and Wolfe (1984).

The demographic composition of the household is also significant in determining the nutritional status of children under three years of age as also in the study of Maxwell *et al.* (2000). Presence of younger and older children above five years in the household worsens the nutritional status of their younger siblings. However, an increase in the percentage of adult females in the household improves the nutritional status of the child which is also found by Sahn (1990). However, the differences are modest, a percentage increase in adult females in the family improves weight of the reference male child by 6.3 g, while one percentage point increase in the children under and above 5 years in the family reduces weight of the reference male child by 4 g and 100 g respectively.

All the variables associated with standard of living or wealth status are significant in determining the nutritional status of the children, as expected (Strauss, 1990 and Horton, 1986). For instance, the coefficient associated with size of the landholding is significantly positive. An increase in size of the landholding by 1 acre would translate into increase of 5 g in the weight of the reference male child.

The impact on weight is greater for housing and amenities. Children living in *pucca* or semi-*pucca* houses have higher weight-for-age z-score than living in *kutcha* houses (Olaniyan, 2002). Living in semi-*pucca* house would improve the weight of the reference male child by 157 g and 337 g if he lives in *pucca* house as compared to *kutcha* house. Similarly, the weight of the reference male child improves by 293 g if he lives in house with electricity as compared to house with no electricity supply.

The source of drinking water is an important factor in determining the nutritional status. In comparison to households using spring, river, pond, rainwater, etc., as source of drinking water, households that use piped water have better nourished children with a difference in the reference weight of 146 g.

Purification of water is equally important. It improves the weight of the reference male child by 122 g as compared to when the household is not purifying water. This is in line with other studies which conclude that safe drinking water reduces the susceptibility to water-borne infections and thus, ensures better nutritional status (Jalan and Ravallion, 2001 and Attanasio *et al.*, 2004).

The provision of healthy environment plays the most crucial role in determining the nutritional status of the children as also found in studies of Esrey *et al.* (1992) and McJunkin (1982). The lack of sanitation can be particular for children under age three in the rural areas, especially as they are weaned and come into contact with possible contaminated food. The weight of the reference male child improves by 358 g, 376 g and 473 g if household is using a public toilet, shared toilet and own toilet respectively, as compared to the situation when the household has no provision of sanitary facility.

7.1.4 The Role of Village-specific Variables

The role of environmental factors is further reinforced by considering drainage facility in the village. The marginal difference of 42 g between weight of the reference male child living in village with open drainage and no drainage system is not statistically significant. Underground drainage is also not significant, probably on account of very few observations (around 1% of the villages that have underground drainage).

Easy access to health facilities implying quick availability of health care facilities would mean better nutritional status of the children. However, the results indicate that there is no significant difference in nutritional status of the children under three years of age who have access to the health facility within the village and those who do not have.

7.2 Correlates of Nutritional Status among Women and Children

In the previous exercise undertaken with reference to nutritional status among children under three years of age, we used the frequency of intakes of certain food items as proxies for the dietary intake variables. In the exercise in this section, we use micronutrient intakes calculated from the NSS consumption data of the households—focusing in particular on iron and vitamins A and C. We also use calorie intake as a direct measure of nutrient intakes. For other determinants, we use a somewhat abbreviated set of environmental factors but a more complete measure of income which is represented by per capita monthly expenditure.

As detailed in section 3.3, this data set is constructed by regional aggregates from the unit record data of both the NSS and NFHS data sets. Consistency checks including the matching of the aggregation at the state level with the published figures ensured that the regional aggregation was performed accurately. The overall sample size is thus 63 regions.

Further, instead of considering only single measure of nutritional status as in the previous section, we consider: (a) the nutritional status of children and adult women jointly; and (b) two distinct measures of nutritional status—anthropometric outcomes and anaemia.

Thus, for anthropometric measures, we use the z-score of weight-for-age of children under the age of three years and body mass index (BMI) for adult women. For the second set of measures, we use the prevalence of anaemia among children below three years and among women as reasoned in section 4.4.2.

Given the multivariate nature of the nutritional status variables, we use canonical correlations to analyse the key relationships (see section 4.4.2). In either case, the explanatory variables are the same. Of particular interest is the relationship between anaemia prevalence and dietary intakes of iron, controlling for exposure to infections as captured by the environmental variables.

The two formulations are:

Percentage of women with BMI less than 18.5, percentage of children who are underweight = f_i (calories, iron, vitamin A, vitamin C, percentage of population having access to sanitation facilities, percentage of population using water purification methods, percentage of population having pump or pipe as source of drinking water and monthly per capita expenditure)

Prevalence of anemia amomg women and prevalence of anaemia among children = f_i (calories, iron, vitamin A, vitamin C, percentage of population having access to sanitation facilities, percentage of population using water purification methods, percentage of population having pump or pipe as source of drinking water, and monthly per capita expenditure)

Before undertaking the canonical correlation analysis, it is important to examine the extent to which the indicators on the right hand side (RHS) are correlated with each other. Table 7.2 presents the correlation matrix which suggests that pair-wise correlations between the right hand side variables may not present a problem for interpreting the canonical covariates. The exceptions are the correlations between calories and micronutrient intakes.

Table 7.2

Correlation Coefficients among Dietary and Non-dietary Variables

Correlation	*Sanitation*	*Pump/pipe*	*Water*	*Calories*	*Iron*	*Vitamin C*	*Vitamin A*	*MPCE*
Sanitation facilities	1							
Pump/pipe	-0.36	1						
Water purification	0.39	-0.32	1					
Calories	0.56	-0.29	0.27	1				
Iron	0.24	-0.27	0.19	0.75	1			
Vitamin C	0.58	-0.12	0.23	0.71	0.38	1		
Vitamin A	0.44	-0.24	0.30	0.79	0.65	0.48	1	
MPCE	0.54	-0.13	0.19	0.29	0.18	0.40	0.13	1

7.2.1 Nutritional Status as Measured by Anthropometric Indicators

The results of canonical correlation between the prevalence of anthropometric failure and set of dietary as well as socioeconomic-environmental variables are laid down in Table 7.3. The first two canonical correlations are 0.86 and 0.44. The F-test values showed that the first canonical correlation is significant (or two sets of variables are related), while second canonical correlation is not significant. Therefore, only the relationship depicted by the first canonical correlation is considered for interpretation.

Table 7.3

Canonical Correlation Coefficients and Variable Loadings (Structural Correlations) for Underweight and Socioeconomic-Dietary Variables

Canonical correlation coefficients	First	Second
Value	**0.86**	0.44
Pr >F	0.00	0.10
Variable	*Structural correlation (loading) for the first canonical*	
Underweight among children	**-0.99**	
Chronic energy deficiency among women	**-0.75**	
Sanitation facilities	**0.80**	
Pump/Pipe	-0.21	
Water purification	0.23	
Calories	**0.42**	
Iron	0.14	
Vitamin C	0.33	
Vitamin A	**0.42**	
Monthly per capita expenditure	**0.89**	

Note: • Bold figures indicate these values are significant[2]

Source: Computed from NSS 55th round and NFHS survey 1998-99

It is to be noted that the two anthropometric variables capture 77 per cent[3] of the variance in the canonical variate representing undernourishment among children and women. As for the canonical variate representing the various socioeconomic-dietary factors (RHS factors), monthly per capita income and sanitary facilities load heavily and negatively on anthropometric failure. Higher the income, lower would be the incidence of underweight among children and women, as is also evident in the recent studies of Attanasio *et al.* (2004) and Block (2002), among others.

Better sanitary conditions would also improve the nutritional status of children and women. Lower intakes of calories and vitamin A load moderately in explaining variation in underweight among children and women, as is also found in Ramakrishnan *et al.* (2004), Demment *et al.* (2003) and Rivera *et al.* (2003). In other words, higher intakes of calories

2. Being equal to or greater than 0.4 as discussed in 4.4.2
3. 0.77=(Sum of square of structural correlations) / 2=$(0.99)^2 + (0.75)^2 / 2$

and vitamin A reduce the prevalence of underweight among children and women. Approximately 57 per cent[4] of the variation in nutritional status variate is determinable from the knowledge of socioeconomic-dietary variables.

It indicates that income, provision of sanitation facilities, intakes of calories and vitamin A are the key variables in determining the undernourishment among children and women. Source and purification of water and iron intakes turn out to be insignificant.

7.2.2 Nutritional Status as Measured by Prevalence of Anaemia

The results of canonical correlation between anaemia—among children and women, and set of dietary and non-dietary factors (RHS)—are put in Table 7.4. Both the correlations are significant as $p<0.0000$. The strength of the linear relationships for the two pairs are 0.77 and 0.68 respectively. In other words, it implies that there exists a significant relationship in nutritional status as measured by prevalence of anaemia and the set of dietary and non-dietary factors.

In the first canonical correlation, nutritional status canonical variate-representing anaemia among women and children—captures 75 per cent[5] of its variance which is average of the square of the canonical correlation. The magnitudes of loadings indicating prevalence of anaemia among women and children is heavily associated with sanitary facilities followed by income, calorie intakes and source of water. Non-availability of sanitary facilities increases the incidence of anaemia among women and children. It is also in accordance with the literature that reports that poor sanitary and hygienic conditions are main source of infection, in particular parasitic infestations that have been important cause of anaemia (WHO, 2000; Gopalan *et al.*, 2000; Bhargava *et al.*, 2001).

Lower monthly per capita expenditure and lower intakes of calories and vitamin C are associated with higher rate of prevalence of anaemia among children and women.

4. 57 per cent is the product of mean squared structure coefficient for a given canonical variable (0.77) times the squared canonical correlation coefficient associated with that canonical variable $(0.86)^2$.

5. $0.75=(-0.93)^2+(0.79)^2 /2$

The second canonical correlation tells us that anaemia among women is particularly associated with poverty and low dietary intake of iron. Therefore, better incomes and higher intakes of calories, iron and vitamin C lower the prevalence of anaemia.

Table 7.4

Canonical Correlation Coefficients and Variable Loadings (Structural Correlations) for Anaemia and Socioeconomic-Dietary Variables

Canonical correlation coefficients	*First*	*Second*
Value	**0.77**	**0.68**
Pr >F	0.0000	0.0000
Variable	*Structural correlation (loading)*	*Structural correlation (loading)*
Anaemia among children	**-0.93**	0.36
Anaemia among women	**-0.79**	**-0.61**
Sanitation facilities	**0.85**	-0.09
Pump/Pipe	**-0.53**	**0.42**
Water purification	**0.45**	-0.09
Calories	**0.55**	0.06
Iron	0.26	**0.37**
Vitamin C	**0.48**	-0.13
Vitamin A	0.28	-0.07
Monthly per capita expenditure	**0.61**	**0.53**

Note: • Bold figures indicate these values are significant[6]

Source: Computed from NSS 55th Round and NFHS Survey 1998-99

Almost half of the variation in prevalence of anaemia among women and children is explained by the RHS canonical variate consisting of socio-economic-dietary variables.[7] Given that this is based on cross-sectional data, this is a fairly high percentage.

6. Being equal to or greater than 0.4 as discussed in 4.4.2
7. The first canonical variate explains 0.75 of nutritional status variate and R^2_1 is 0.59. Hence, optimal knowledge of socio-dietary-environmental variables explains 0.44=(0.75*0.59) of the variance of anaemia. Similarly, the second canonical variate explains 0.25 of nutritional status variate and R^2_2 is 0.46. Therefore, optimal knowledge of socio-dietary-environmental variables explains 0.04=(0.25*0.46) of the variance in anaemia. Together it explains 0.48=(0.44+0.04) of the variance in anaemia among women and children.

7.3 A Summary of the Main Results

Using NFHS (1998-99) survey data, we have examined the effect of nutrient intake and socioeconomic-environmental factors on weight-for-age of children under three years of age for rural India. These factors have been classified into child, parent, household or village specific factors. The significance of these variables has been assessed in terms of significance of t-ratios or changes in weight of the underweight male child who is nine months old.

It has been found that intra-household demographic factors like birth order or age of the child are the most important factors influencing the nutritional status of the children. It is the intra-household competition for resources and care that affects health outcome of the child significantly.

The condition of living environment followed by the socioeconomic status of the household are other variables which have significant influence on the health outcome of the children. Availability of effective sanitation, water and housing facilities are the key factors that comprise the living environment for a household. It stresses the importance of hygienic conditions in positively determining the growth of the children as it reduces the risk and spread of infections due to bacteria, viruses and helminthes which would otherwise result into the poor nutritional status. Better quality of house, electricity connection and possession of land as an economic asset improves the weight-for-age of the child.

The social status of mother, primary caregiver, in terms of occupation and autonomy, are also most important in determining nutritional status of preschool children.

Strong familial bond and greater autonomy of mother in household decision-making considerably enhance the nutritional status of the children under three years of age. Young and better nourished mothers are able to improve the nutritional status of the children right from the weight at birth to upbringing of the child later on.

Dietary intake variables are significant but their effect is lower in magnitude as compared to demographic and living environment variables. Among dietary factors, quality of complementary food appears to be the more significant variable than breastfeeding for the children of age under three years. It highlights the role of green leafy vegetables and fruits, which are rich sources of vitamins and minerals, in determining the nutritional status of children under the age of three years.

A similar result is obtained with the data set that relates nutrient intakes, social, economic and environmental indicators to the nutritional status of women and children at the regional level in the second exercise. Among the nutrient intakes besides calories, vitamin A appears to be significant in determining the prevalence of underweight; iron and vitamin C explain cross-sectional variations in anaemia prevalence.

These results indicate that an adequate nutrient intake is only one of the factors, while living environment and other social factors, in addition to independent effects of income, emerge as more powerful variables in determining nutritional status of an individual.

8 Conclusions

During the last two decades, a sea change has occurred in the understanding of the problem of malnutrition. Malnutrition is no longer limited to food security based on per capita calorie availability. It now encompasses the more comprehensive concept of nutritional security where the outcome is not merely freedom from hunger but freedom from ill health.

Since 1947, with the objective of reducing poverty and hunger, India undertook systematic planning with a focus on agricultural and industrial development. By the turn of the century, it recorded success in poverty reduction, improvement in the health in terms of decline in mortality rate and fertility rate, and increase in life expectancy. India's foodgrain production went up from 50 million tonnes in 1950-51 to over 200 million tonnes in 1999-2000—a four-fold increase. The population during the same period increased from 350 million to 1 billion. Thus, the growth in foodgrain production surpassed population growth, and India emerged as a country with enough food reserves to provide some degree of national food security.

In spite of this success story, some worrisome aspects with regard to malnutrition, whether measured in terms of nutrient inadequacies or anthropometric failures, remain. Almost half of the children under the age of three years are still underweight and stunted. It is estimated that about one-third of neonates weigh less than 2.5 kg, and no major reduction in the proportion of low birth weight babies is reported. A disproportionately large proportion of women and children remain malnourished. The prevalence of anaemia in the general population in India is among the highest in the world, with 50-90 per cent of pregnant women being anaemic.

These figures point to the need of addressing a form of hunger—of vitamins and minerals—that remains silent or unnoticed and thus, hidden. The nature and extent of damage caused by deficiencies of these micronutrients (vitamins and minerals) has serious repercussions on child growth and development, cognitive skills, intelligence, mental acuity and productivity levels.

WHO estimates of the magnitude of micronutrient malnutrition indicate that the total number of people at risk of one or more of the deficiencies is around 2 billion, most of whom live in developing countries. In India alone, more than 300 million people are affected by one or more of the micronutrient deficiencies (Mannar, 2004).

Against this backdrop, the present study examines important issues related to malnutrition in rural India. The objectives of this research work are to:

- Provide estimates of the quantum of intake of, as well as deprivation in, macronutrients (calorie, protein, fat) and micronutrients (vitamin A, vitamin B [thiamine, niacin, riboflavin], vitamin C and iron) in rural India and among 15 major states;
- Examine how the macro and micronutrient intakes vary with income, and how these are conditioned by education, occupational structure, household size and composition, seasonality, social status; and
- Examine how the nutritional status of children under the age of three years (weight-for-age) varies with the nutrient intake levels, socio–economic variables and environmental factors. Besides, the study also identifies the key factors that are associated with prevalence of underweight and anaemia among women in the age 15-49 years and children under the age of 3 years.

The two data sets used in this study are the all India surveys on consumer expenditure conducted by the National Sample Survey Organisation (NSSO) in 1983 and 1999-2000 and National Family Health Survey (NFHS) in 1998-99 for rural India. The NFHS collects detailed information from ever-married woman between 15-49 years and their children under the age of 3 years.

8.1 Results on Nutrient Deprivation

In rural India, we find that diets have diversified. Over time, the share of cereals in total food expenditure has declined, while that of milk, meat, vegetables and fruits has increased. This shift in the tastes has translated into a decline of almost 2 kg in cereal consumption per capita per month between 1983 and 1999-2000. What is more important is that this substitution from cereals to non-cereals has not only occurred among the rich, but also among the poor. Further, there has been a doubling in the dietary diversity index (DDI) over this period.

This trend in diversification should have implied improvements in micronutrient intakes. However, this has not been the case. In comparison to 1983, there has been a decline in the average intake of most nutrients (with the exception of vitamin C and fat) in terms of head count ratio (HCR) of micronutrient deprivation. Thus, the situation with respect to nutrient intakes appears to be worsening. Also, even though the availability of vitamin C and fat has increased over time, HCRs of nutrient deprivation are as high as 44 per cent and 71 per cent respectively. It is only in the case of thiamine and niacin that the head count percentage of deprivation is relatively low, at about 10 per cent and 15 per cent respectively. However, the Foster-Greer-Thorbecke FGT (1) and FGT (2) measures are indicative of an improvement in the depth and severity of nutrient inadequacy in all nutrients except iron for rural India.

Not surprisingly, deprivation levels for all the nutrients are much higher among the poor than among the rich. What is intriguing is that nutrient deprivation has increased over time, not just among the poorest, but also among the richest 25 per cent (except vitamin A), although the depth and severity of the gap has decreased.

The increase in HCR of iron deprivation is particularly dramatic, with nearly all those belonging to the poorest expenditure group having deficient intakes of iron, and as many as three-fifths of the richest 25 per cent having below recommended dietary allowance (RDA) intakes. Also, despite the fall in vitamin C deprivation, one-fifth of the richest quartile have inadequate intakes—this is unexpected, given that this group is not constrained by income and could afford a nutrient-sufficient diet.

In general, levels of deprivation are much lower in the states of Haryana, Himachal Pradesh, Rajasthan, Punjab and Uttar Pradesh than in Andhra Pradesh, Gujarat, Karnataka, Kerala, Maharashtra, Tamil Nadu, Bihar, Madhya Pradesh, Orissa and West Bengal. Andhra Pradesh, Madhya

Pradesh, Maharashtra, Karnataka and Tamil Nadu are the few states which have deteriorated in terms of nutritional deprivation for most of the nutrients across all income groups.

Broadly speaking, except vitamin C and fat, there has been an increase in the incidence of nutrient deficiency in most of the states. The percentage of population getting less than the RDA of protein, riboflavin and iron has increased in almost all states. The evidence for niacin and vitamin A is mixed, with half of the states witnessing an increase in the level of deficiency and the other half witnessing a decline.

Focusing on the poorest quartile of different states, the pattern is broadly the same, the exceptions being the poorer states of Kerala, West Bengal, Orissa and Bihar which experienced a decrease in HCR of nutrient deprivation.

This worsening trend in micronutrient intakes is, at first, surprising, given the diversification in diets. However, diversification has implied lower cereal intakes, and cereals account for almost three-fourths of the intake of these nutrients except vitamin A. Thus, this decline explains virtually all of the decreased nutrient intakes observed. While there has been increased consumption of other commodities such as vegetables, fruits, milk, meat and so on, these have not been of sufficiently high orders of magnitude to offset the consequences of reduced cereal intakes. As far as vitamin A is concerned, though it is primarily sourced in vegetables and fruits, its intake has decreased primarily on account of an apparent decrease in the consumption of green leafy vegetables.

Nutritional status also depends on bioavailability. The increase in the intakes of vitamin C and fat is significant, as both are important in enhancing the bioavailability of many micronutrients, especially iron, thiamine and vitamin A. Thus, at least for iron, improved bioavailability could mitigate the decline in intakes to some extent.

Turning to nutritional status, one finds a weak correlation between nutrient intakes and nutritional status at least at the state level. For example, the southern states—Kerala, Tamil Nadu and Andhra Pradesh—have lower calorie intakes, but also have lower prevalence of underweight children. Andhra Pradesh, Madhya Pradesh, Maharashtra, Karnataka and

Tamil Nadu have seen a worsening of deprivation in intakes for most of the nutrients irrespective of income groups. This is apparently a paradox, for if we look at the nutritional status as measured in terms of anthropometric measures or anaemia, we find that these states rank high in terms of health outcomes. The average iron intake in Tamil Nadu and Kerala is lower than the RDA, yet these states do not have a high prevalence of anaemia among women and preschool children as compared to Punjab and Haryana.

Similarly, the relationship between income and nutritional status is also not strong. States with high prevalence rates of anaemia among children and among women include richer states such as Punjab and Haryana, as well as the poor states of Bihar and Orissa. Analysing the determinants of nutrient intakes and nutritional status provides some insight into the problem, though not a resolution.

8.2 Results on Correlates of Nutrient Intakes

The role of various factors in determining the demand for nutrient intakes has been explored through estimation of nutrient demand functions. Nutrient demand functions for nine macro and micronutrients have been estimated as functions of income, and demographic, socioeconomic and other variables, using seemingly unrelated regression (SUR). The results suggest that there is a clear distinction to be made between the micronutrients (vitamin A and vitamin C which are sourced primarily in non-cereal foods, and the rest of the micronutrients.

Income elasticities of nutrient demand are positive, though typically below one. They vary significantly by income and are high for the poorest quartile. So income is an important determinant of nutrient intakes, especially for the poor. This is true of all macro and micronutrients. Elasticities for vitamin A, vitamin C and fat are higher than those for calories. For thiamine, riboflavin, niacin and protein, the magnitude of elasticities is almost the same as for calories.

On an average, these nutrient-expenditure elasticities have declined over time except for micronutrients that are sourced in non-staple foods—vitamin A, vitamin C and fat. This decline can be discerned in almost all the states except in some of the Bihar, Madhya Pradesh, Rajasthan and Uttar Pradesh (BIMARU) (poor) states plus Andhra Pradesh and Maharashtra.

However, for the poorest quartile, nutrient-expenditure elasticities have increased in many more states.

The evidence does not indicate seasonality in nutrient deprivation to any appreciable degree except in the case of vitamin C and vitamin A, where the greater availability of seasonal fruits and vegetables during the cooler months of January-March results in higher intakes in majority of the states. So seasonality is an issue only for vitamins A and C.

Demographic factors significantly influence nutrient intakes. As far as household composition is concerned, a higher proportion of children in the household is associated with lower per capita intakes of cereal-sourced nutrients in most states, as one might expect. However, the proportion of adult females in the household does not affect the per capita intakes of nutrients; for many micronutrients, the requirements for adult women do differ significantly from those of adult men. The only exception is in the case of iron where the coefficient is negative and significant. This is of particular concern because of the skewed distribution of iron requirements for women.

There is no significant difference in intakes of most of the nutrients between households self-employed in agriculture and agricultural labour households, a somewhat unexpected result.

Also, controlling for other factors, scheduled caste (SC) or scheduled tribe (ST) households have lower fat intakes as compared to other households, while no significant difference emerges for other nutrient intakes in majority of the states.

Somewhat surprisingly, the coefficient associated with literacy turns out to be perverse for most states in the case of calories, protein, thiamine, riboflavin, niacin and iron. It is insignificant in the case of vitamins A and C. While the insignificant signs may be explained by the observation that dietary habits are dictated largely by tradition, and are unlikely to be influenced by the nutritional knowledge that literacy may engender, this cannot explain the perverse sign. Clearly, this is an issue that needs to be explored further.

No significant difference in nutrient intakes of female-headed and male-headed households is observed.

8.3 Results on Correlates of Nutritional Status

For examining the determinants of nutritional status, two separate exercises have been undertaken. In the first exercise, we use a fixed effects specification to model the determinants of the nutritional status of rural children under the age of three years using unit record data from NFHS (1998-99). Standardised weight-for-age z-score is used as an indicator of nutritional status of children under the age of three years as it measures both acute as well as chronically malnourished or deprived in health care. The explanatory variables are defined at the child, parent, household and village levels, ranging from age and gender at the individual level to the availability of health facilities at the community level.

In second exercise, we exploit the near-coincidence of the NSS survey in 1999-2000 and the NFHS survey in 1998-99 and construct a data set with the NSS region as the unit of observation for rural India. We use two important indicators of nutritional status, namely, the prevalence of anthropometric failure and prevalence of anaemia among mothers and children. We have clubbed the nutritional status for mothers and children together to represent different sets of nutritional status indicators; however, one has to remember that these are cross-sectional data, with region-specific aggregates of health status. We try to identify associations between nutritional status and nutrient intake and socioeconomic variables with the help of canonical correlations using this cross-section data set. This technique helps us in identifying the components of one set of variables that are most highly related (linearly) to the components of the other set of variables.

The results of the first exercise suggest that among the child-specific factors, birth order of the child has substantial effect on the weight-for-age. Higher birth order is a disadvantage for nutritional outcomes among young children. Further, the quality of complementary food appears to be more significant than breastfeeding.

Among the parent-specific variables, the role of the mother is found to be more crucial than that of the father in determining the weight-for-age of the preschool child. Mothers who exercise autonomy in household decision making enhance the nutritional status of their children under three years of age. However, contrary to expectations, higher education among mothers does not appear to improve nutritional status. Finally, better nourished mothers have better nourished children.

Provision of safe drinking water, sanitation facilities and type of house are the household-specific variables that appear to be more significant than other living environmental variables in determining the nutritional status of children. This underscores the importance of hygienic conditions that reduce the risk and spread of infections, as infections are a prime cause of ill health among children. The effects of wealth variables as represented by provision of electricity and size of land holding are not as strong as those of environmental factors.

Further, larger-sized households have better nourished children, though the effect is marginal. Household composition variables are significant but have a smaller impact on weight-for-age as compared to economic and environmental variables. A larger proportion of women in a household is associated with better nutritional status of children. This may perhaps reflect the better caring abilities of women as compared to men. The deleterious effect of a larger proportion of children in the family indicates that children compete for limited household resources.

The existence of drainage facility and health facility in the village have a positive but statistically insignificant impact on the nutritional status of the children.

The analysis of the nutritional status production function thus highlights the role of demographic factors like birth order and age as the most important factors followed by condition of living environment and economic status of the household in determining the nutritional status. Dietary intake variables are significant but their effect is lower in magnitude as compared to demographic and living environment variables.

A similar result is obtained in the second exercise with the data set that relates nutrient intakes, social, economic and environmental indicators to the nutritional status of women and children at the regional level.

The prevalence of underweight is more strongly associated with income and provision of sanitation facilities followed by nutrient intakes—calories and vitamin A. Quality of water and iron intake do not appear to be significant in explaining underweight among women and children.

As in case of anthropometric failure, the prevalence of anaemia is strongly associated with income and provision of sanitation facilities but, here, quality of water appears to be significant. Among the nutrient intakes, besides calories, iron and vitamin C explain cross-sectional variations in anaemia.

It is important to note here that while ideally, such relationships are best tested using community level data, the use of aggregate data has its own advantage, in that it is nationally representative and the conclusions have wider applicability than may be possible with community studies.

These results suggest that while it is necessary to track trends in micronutrient intakes and dietary diversity, nutritional status is also influenced by a clean living environment and intra-household demographics, in addition to the independent effects of income. Thus, public health interventions need to take a more comprehensive view of factors that lead to positive health outcomes.

8.4 Policy Implications

This study has made an attempt to quantify malnutrition in rural India in terms of nutritional inadequacies, with a focus on micronutrients, and to appreciate the complexity of its determinants. Although the NSS and NFHS are rich data sets, a more comprehensive analysis of the relationship between nutritional status and nutrient intakes and other factors would necessitate the use of a data set for which the unit of observation is an individual and has information both with respect to intakes and outcomes. Such data sets are, however, rarely nationally representative. Despite the limitations placed by the use of these data sets, several findings of this research are robust to the choice of data set and method used, and have significant implications for policy.

The nutritional status of the rural Indian population is quite poor, whether looked at from point of view of prevalence of micronutrient deprivation or anthropometric indicators. The extent of dietary diversification registered between 1983 and 1999-2000 has not been of a sufficient order of magnitude to reduce undernourishment. Rather, it would appear that micronutrient intakes have worsened as a consequence.

Therefore, dietary diversification alone cannot be relied upon to alleviate micronutrient deficiencies, at least in the near future.

The analysis conducted has revealed that while ensuring adequate nutrient intakes is important, the role of sanitation factors within the household and intra-household demographics is stronger than may have been expected. Thus, improvements in the availability of a clean living environment can produce dramatic improvements in nutritional status.

Indeed, water can itself be viewed as a nutrient; improvement in the quality and quantity of its provision can bring desired results in the nutritional status. This may necessitate appropriate investment in toilets, and other sanitation infrastructure, and provision of potable water at the community level. Government policies need to be geared to this as a high priority. However, what is also necessary is community participation and sanitation education programmes to foster widespread behavioural change.

This is not to suggest that the role of income is unimportant, or that the results are supportive of growth pessimism. Our results show that income is a significant determinant of both nutrient intakes and nutritional outcomes. Thus, interventions geared at increasing the disposable household income would positively affect nutrient demand and nutritional status. This could include both direct interventions like cash transfers, wage employment programmes, targeted price subsidies or other poverty alleviation programmes. But ensuring income growth alone may not be sufficient to alleviate undernourishment.

Also crucial are intra-household demographics and the status of primary caregiver. It is perhaps the interstate differences in all these parameters that may explain the paradox of low micronutrient intakes and better nutritional status among the southern Indian states. These findings suggest that, in addition, programmes to raise social awareness about strong familial bonds, empowerment of women, improvement in quality of complementary diet, promotion of breast feeding, family planning programmes (to address the problems of later-born siblings), are all measures that can help in the improvement of the nutritional status of children.

The realisation of these goals could be possible if concerted efforts are initiated at national level along with state level thrust, as there are substantial interstate variations in nutritional status of the population.

Clearly, there is no single solution to the problem of micronutrient malnutrition; what is required is a set of complementary strategies. A key is a change in mindsets so as to focus more on improving sanitation and drinking water supplies, in addition to other strategies for augmenting nutrient intakes, including income enhancement, behaviour-change communication, nutrition education and supplementation or fortification efforts. A thrust should be put on creating nutritional awareness among people, especially mothers, than simply imparting formal education. Nutritional awareness programme is a *sine qua non* to bring about the desired change. It is clear that these need to be undertaken on a war footing if substantial reductions in micronutrient malnutrition are to be achieved. To achieve the millennium development goals, a veritable nutrition revolution is necessary.

Bibliography

Acharya, S.S. (1989). *Socioeconomic Impact of 1987 Drought in Rajasthan*. Jaipur: Department of Agricultural Economics. Rajasthan Agricultural University.

ACC/SCN (2000). "Low birthweight", *Nutrition Policy Paper 18*. September. United Nations.

Alderman, H. (1990). "Nutritional status in Ghana and its determinants", *Policy Analysis Working Paper 3*. Washington DC.

Anderson, M.A. (1981). "Health and nutrition impact of potable water in rural Bolivia", *Journal of Tropical Pediatrics* 27(1): 39-46.

Askew, E.W. (1995). "Environmental and physical stress and nutritional requirements", *American Journal of Clinical Nutrition* 61: 631-37.

Asobayire, F.S., P. Adou, L. Davidsson, J.D. Cook and R.F. Hurrell (2001). "Prevalence of iron deficiency, with and without concurrent anemia, in population groups with high prevalence of malaria and other infections: a study in Côte d'Ivoire", *American Journal of Clinical Nutrition* 74: 776–82.

Attanasio, O., L.C. Gómez and A. Gómez (2004). "Child health in rural Colombia: Determinants and policy interventions", *Economics and Human Biology* 2(3): 411-38.

Bairagi, R. (1986). "Effects of bias and random error in anthropometry and in age on estimation of malnutrition", *American Journal of Epidemiology* 123(1): 185-91.

Bajpai, N., J.D. Sachs and N. Volavka (2005). "India's challenge to meet the millennium development goals", *CGSD Working Paper* No. 24.

Baltagi, B.H. (1995). *Econometric Analysis of Panel Data*. New York: John Wiley and Sons.

Barber, S. and P. Gertler (2001). "Child health and the quality of medical care", *(Mimeo)*.

Barr, S.I., Suzanne P. Murphy, Tanya D. Agurs-Collins and Mary I. Poos (2003). "Planning diets for individuals using the dietary reference intakes", *Nutrition Reviews* 61(10): 352-60.

Barrera, A. (1990). "The role of maternal education and its interaction with public health programs in child health production", *Journal of Development Economics* 32(1): 69-91.

Beard, J. (2001). "Functional consequences of nutritional anemia in adults", in U. Ramakrishnan (ed.), *Nutritional Anemias*. Fla., USA: CRC Press.

Behrman, J.R. (1988a). "Nutrition, health, birth order and seasonality: Intrahousehold allocation in rural India", *Journal of Development Economics*: 43-62, February 28.

———. (1988b). "Intrahousehold allocation of nutrients in rural India: Are boys favored? Do parents exhibit inequality aversion?", *Oxford Economic Papers* 40(1): 32-54, March. Oxford University Press.

———. (1988c). "Nutrition and incomes: Tightly wedded or loosely meshed?" Pew/Cornell Lecture Series on *Food and Nutrition Policy*. Ithaca: Cornell University.

Behrman, J.R. and A.B. Deolalikar (1987). "Will developing country nutrition improve with income? A case study for rural south India", *Journal of Political Economy* 95(3): 492-507.

———. (1988). "Health and nutrition", in J.R. Behrman and T.N.Srinivasan, (eds.), *Handbook of Development Economics* 1: 631-711. Amsterdam: North-Holland.

Behrman, J.R. and B.L. Wolfe (1984). "More evidence on nutrition demand: income seems overrated and women's schooling underemphasized", *Journal of Development Economics* 14: 105-28.

———. (1987). "How does mothers' schooling affect family health, nutrition, medical-care usage and household sanitation", *Journal of Econometrics* 36: 185-204.

Behrman, J.R. and E. Skoufias (2004). "Correlates and determinants of child anthropometrics in Latin America: Background and overview of the symposium", *Economics and Human Biology* 2(3): 335-51.

Bennett, M.K. (1954). *The World's Food: A Study of the Interrelations of World Population, National Diets and Food Potentials*. New York: Harper & Brothers.

Bernstein, I.H., C. Garbin, and G. Teng (1988). *Applied multivariate analysis*. New York: Springer Verlag.

Bhalotra, S. and C.L. Atfield (1998). "Intrahousehold resource allocation in rural Pakistan: A semi-parametric analysis", *Journal of Applied Econometrics* 13(5): 463-80.

Bhargava, A. (1991a). "Estimating short and long run income elasticities of foods and nutrients for rural south India", *Journal of Royal Statistical Society* 154: 157-74.

———. (1991b). "Identification and panel data models with endogenous resources", *Review of Economic Studies* 58: 129-40.

———. (2001). "Nutrition, health, and economic development: Some policy priorities", *Food Nutrition Bulletin* 22(2): 173–78.

Bhargava, A., H.E. Bouis and N.S. Scrimshaw (2001). "Dietary intakes and socioeconomic factors are associated with the hemoglobin concentration of Bangladeshi women", *Journal of Nutrition* 131: 758-64.

Bhargava, A. and Melanie Fox-Kean (2003). "The effects of maternal education versus cognitive test scores on child nutrition in Kenya", *Economics and Human Biology* 1(3): 309–19.

Bidinger, P.D., T.S. Walker, B. Sarkar, A.R. Murthy and P. Babu (1990). "Economic, health and nutritional consequences of the mid-1980s drought on a tank irrigated, deccan village in south India", *Progress Report* 98. ICRISAT, Hyderabad: Resource Management Programme, Economics Group.

Block, S. (2002). "Nutrition knowledge versus schooling in the demand for child micronutrient status", *Food Policy and Applied Nutrition Program, Discussion Paper* No. 10. The Gerald J. and Dorothy K. Friedman School of Nutrition Science and Policy, Tufts University.

Bouis, H.E. (1990). "Evaluating demand for calories for urban and rural populations in the Philippines: Implications for nutrition policy under economic recovery", *World Development* 18(2): 281-99.

———. (1994). "The effect of income on demand for food in poor countries: Are our food consumption databases giving us reliable estimates?", *Journal of Development Economics* 44: 199-226.

Bouis, H.E. and L.J. Haddad (1992). "Are estimates of calorie-income elasticities too high?", *Journal of Development Economics* 39: 333-64.

Bouis, H.E. and M.J. Novenario-Reese (1997). "The determinants of demand for micronutrients: An analysis of rural households in Bangladesh," Food Consumption and Nutrition Division, *Discussion Paper* No. 32. Washington DC: International Food Policy Research Institute.

Briscoe, J. (1979). "The quantitative effect of infection on the use of food by young children in poor countries", *American Journal of Clinical Nutrition* 32: 648-76.

Brooker, S., N. Peshu, P.A. Warn, M. Mosobo, H.L. Guyatt, K. Marsh and R.W. Snow (1999). "The epidemiology of hookworm infection and its contribution to anaemia among pre-school children on the Kenyan coast", *Trans. Royal Society of Tropical Medicine and Hygiene* 93: 240-46.

Carpenter, C.E. and A.W. Mahoney (1992). "Contributions of heme and nonheme iron to human nutrition", *Critical Reviews in Food Science Nutrition* 31: 333-67.

Cebu Study Team (1991). "Underlying and proximate determinants of child health: The Cebu longitudinal health and nutrition study", *American Journal of Epidemiology* 133(2): 185-201.

———. (1992). "A child health production function estimated from longitudinal data", *Journal of Development Economics* 38: 323-51.

Cervantes, S., S. Salazer and Z. Rojas (1981). "Socio-economic characteristics of functional groups of the malnourished population in Costa Rica", *UNICEF Social Statistical Bulletin* 4(4): 1-9.

Chandra, R.K. (1979). "Prospective studies of the effect of breast feeding on incidence of infection and allergy," *Acta Paediatr. Scand.* 68: 691-94.

Chandrasekhar, C.P. and Jayati Ghosh (2003). "The calorie consumption puzzle", *Financial Daily*, The Hindu group of publications. February 11.

Checkley, W., R.H. Gilman, R.E. Black, L.D. Epstein, L. Cabrera, C.R. Sterling and L.H. Moulton (2004). "Effect of water and sanitation on childhood health in a poor Peruvian Peri-Urban community", *The Lancet* 363: 112-18.

Chelliah, J.R. and R. Sudershan (1999). *Income, Poverty and Beyond: Human Development in India*. Social Science Press.

Chen, C. and N.S. Scrimshaw (1983). *Diarrhea and Malnutrition: Interactions Mechanisms and Interventions*. New York: Plenum Press.

Chernichovsky, D. and A.A. Kielmann (1977). "Correlates of preschool child growth in rural Punjab", in A.A. Kielmann, C.E. Taylor and R.L. Parker (eds.), *The Narangwal Nutrition Study, (Mimeo)*.

Clark, Carol A.M. (1981). "Demographic and socio-economic correlates of infant growth in Guatemala", *Rand Corporation Report*, N-1702-AID/RF.

Dasgupta, P. (1993). *An Inquiry into Well-being and Destitution*. Oxford, Clarendon Press.

Datt, G., Martin Ravallion. and Valerie Kozel (2003). "A model based assessment on India's progress in reducing poverty in the 1990s", *Economic and Political Weekly* 38(4): 355-61.

Deaton, A. (1997). *The Analysis of Household Surveys: A Microeconometric Approach*, World Bank, Washington DC: Johns Hopkins University Press.

———. (2003a). "Prices and poverty in India, 1987-2000", *Economic and Political Weekly* 38(4): 362-68.

———. (2003b). "Adjusted Indian poverty estimates for 1999-2000", *Economic and Political Weekly* 38(4): 322-26.

Deaton, A. and C. Paxon (1998). "Economies of scale, household size and the demand for food", *Journal of Political Economy* 106: 898-930

Deaton, A. and J. Dreze (2002). "Poverty and inequality in India–A re-examination", *Economic and Political Weekly* 36: 3729-748. September 7.

Delgado, M. and Peter Robinson (1992). "Nonparametric and semiparametric methods for economic research", *Journal of Economic Surveys* 6(3): 201-49.

Demment, M.W., M.M. Young and R.L. Sensenig (2003). "Providing micronutrients through food-based solutions: A key to human and national development", *Journal of Nutrition. Supplement: Animal Source Foods to Improve Micronutrient Nutrition in Developing Countries* 133: 3879S-3885S. November.

Desai, P., K.L Standard, W.E. Miall (1970). "Socio-economic and cultural influences on child growth in rural Jamaica", *Journal of Biosocial Science* (2): 133-43.

Duflo, E. (2000). "Child health and household resources in South Africa: Evidence from the old age pension program", *American Economic Review* 90(2): 393-98.

Engle, P., P. Menon and L. Haddad (1999). "Care and nutrition: Concepts and measurement", *World Development* 27(8): 1309–337.

Esrey, S.A. (1996). "Waste, water and well-being: a multicountry study", *American Journal of Epidemiology* 143: 608-23.

Esrey, S.A., J.P. Habicht and G. Casella (1992). "The complementary effect of latrines and increased water usage on the growth of infants in rural Lesotho", *American Journal of Epidemiology* 135: 659-66.

Eveleth, P.B. and J.M. Tanner (1976, 1990). *Worldwide Variation in Human Growth*. New York: Cambridge University Press.

FAO (occasional, 1996). *World Food Survey*. Rome: Food and Agricultural Organisation.

Ferguson, D.M., L.J. Horwood, F.T. Shannon and B. Taylor (1981). "Breast-feeding, gastrointestinal and lower respiratory illness in the first two years," *Australian Paediatric Journal* 17: 191-95.

Foster, J., J.Greer and E.Thorbecke (1984). "A class of decomposable poverty measures", *Econometrica* 52: 761-65.

Girma, W. and T. Genebo (2002). *Determinants of Nutritional Status of Women and Children in Ethiopia*. Maryland, USA: ORC Macro: Calverton.

Gibson, J. and Scott Rozelle (2002). "How elastic is calorie demand? Parametric, nonparametric and semiparametric results for urban Papua New Guinea", *Journal of Development Studies* 38 (6): 23-46.

Genebo, T., W. Girma, J. Hadir and T. Demmissie (1999). "The association of children's nutritional status to maternal education in Ziggbaboto, Guragie Zone South Ethiopia", *Ethiopian Journal of Health Development* 13(1): 55-61.

Gopalan, C. (1995). "Towards food and nutritional security", *Economic and Political Weekly* 30(52): 134-41.

———. (2004). "India's food production policies: Need for nutrition orientation", *Nutritional Foundation of India Bulletin* 25(3).

Gopalan, C., B.V.R. Sastry and S.C. Balasubramanian (2000). *Nutritive Value of Indian Foods*. Hyderabad, India: National Institute of Nutrition.

———. (2004). *Nutritive Value of Indian Foods*. Hyderabad: National Institute of Nutrition.

Greiner, T. and M.C. Latham (1981). "Factors associated with nutritional status among young children in St. Vincent", *Ecology of Food Nutrition* 10: 135-41.

Gross, R., G. Lopez de Romaña and J. Tomaro (2000). "A life-cycle approach to multi-micronutrient supplementation: Rationale and programme concept", *Food Nutrition Bulletin* 21: 270–74.

Guilkey, D.K. and J.F. Stewart (1995). "Infant feeding patterns and the marketing of infant foods in the Philippines", *Economic Development and Cultural Change* 43(2): 369–99.

Haddad, L. (1987). "Agricultural household modeling with intrahousehold food distribution: A case study of commercialization in a southern Philippine Province", *Ph.D Dissertation*. California, Stanford University: Food Research Institute.

Haddad, L. and H. Alderman (1997). *Intrahousehold Resource Allocation in Developing Countries: Models, Methods, and Policy*. Baltimore: Johns Hopkins University Press.

Haddad, L., S. Bhattarai, M. Immink and S. Kumar (1996). "Managing interactions between household food security and preschooler health", *Food, Agriculture and the Environment Discussion Paper No.16*. Washington, DC: International Food Policy Research Institute.

Hebert, J.R. (1985). "Effects of components of sanitation on nutritional status: findings from South Indian settlements", *International Journal of Epidemiology* 14(1): 143-52.

Henry, F.J. (1981). "Environmental sanitation infection and nutritional status of rural St. Lucia, West Indies", *Trans. Royal Society of Tropical Medicine and Hygiene* 75(4): 507-13.

Hobcraft, J. (2000). "The consequences of female empowerment for child well-being: A review of concepts, issues, and evidence in a post-Cairo context", in H. Presser and G. Sen (ed.), *Women's empowerment and demographic processes*. Oxford University Press.

Horton, S. (1986). "Child nutrition and family size in the Philippines", *Journal of Development Economics* 23(1): 161-76.

———. (1988). "Birth order and child nutritional status: Evidence from the Philippines", *Economic Development and Cultural Change* 36(2): 341-45.

IIPS and ORC Macro (1992-93). *National Family Health Survey (NFHS-1), 1992–93*. Mumbai: IIPS.

International Conference on Nutrition (ICS) (1993). *Plan of Action for Nutrition*. Rome: FAO.

International Nutritional Anemia Consultative Group (2002). *Anemia, Iron Deficiency, and Iron Deficiency Anemia*, USA: INACG publications.

Jalan, J. and M. Ravallion (2001). "Does piped water reduce diarrhoeal disease for children in rural India", *Working Paper No. 2664*. Washington DC, USA.

James, W.P.T., A. Ferro-Luzzi and J.C. Waterlow (1988), "Definition of chronic energy deficiency in adults", *European Journal of Clinical Nutrition* 42: 969-81.

Jha, R. (2003). "The spatial distribution of calorie deficiency in rural India in the last three quinquennial rounds of NSS", *Working Paper*. Division of Economics, Research School of Pacific and Asian Studies, Australian National University.

Jurgens, H.W., I.A. Aune and U. Pieper (1990). *International Data on Anthropometry, Occupational Safety and Health Series* 65. Geneva: International Labour Office.

Judge, G.G., R.C. Hill, W.E. Griffiths, H. Lutkepehl and Tsoung-Chao Lee (1988). *Introducation to the Theory and Practice of Econometrics*. John Wiley and Sons.

Kennedy, E.T. and B. Cogill (1987). "Income and nutrition effect of commercialisation of agriculture in south-western Kenya", *Research Report* No. 63. Washington DC: International Food Policy Research Institute.

Kumar, P. and V.C. Mathur (1996). "Structural changes in demand for food in India", *Indian Journal of Agriculture Economics* 51(4): 664-73.

Laessig, R.E. and E.J. Duckett (1979). "Canonical correlation analysis: Potential for environmental health planning", *American Journal of Public Health* 69: 353-59.

Lancaster, G., P. Maitra and R. Ray (2004). "Gender bias in nutrient intake: Evidence from selected Indian states", *(Mimeographed)*. Australia: Department of Economics, Monash University, Australian Research Council.

Lancaster, Kelvin (1971). *Consumer Demand—A New Approach*. New York and London: Columbia University Press.

Lavy, V., J. Strauss and P. de Vreyer (1996). "Quality of health care, survival, and health outcomes in Ghana", *Journal of Health Economics* 15(3): 333-57.

Leslie, J. (1998). "Women's work and child nutrition in the third world", *World Development* 16(11): 1341–362.

Lipton, M. (1983). "Poverty, undernutrition and hunger", *World Bank Staff Working Paper* No. 597. World Bank.

Magnani, R.J., D.C. Clay, A.L. Adlakha, S.C. Tourkin (1985). *Breastfeeding, Water/ Sanitation, and Childhood Nutrition in the Phillippine, (Mimeo)*.

Mannar, M.G. Venkatesh (2004). "Micronutrient deficiencies and hidden hunger", in M.S. Swaminathan and Pedro Medrano (eds.), *Towards Hunger Free India-From Vision to Action*. Chennai, India: East West Books.

Martorell, R., C. Yarbrough, S. Yarbrough and R.E. Klein (1980). "The impact of ordinary illnesses on the dietary intakes of malnourished children", *American Journal of Clinical Nutrition* 33: 345-50.

Martorell, R. and T.J. Ho (1984). "Malnutrition, morbidity and mortality," in *Population and Development Review* 10: 49-68.

Martorell, R., J. Leslie and P.R. Moock (1984). "Characteristics and determinants of child nutritional status in Nepal", *American Journal of Clinical Nutrition* 39: 74-86.

Martorell, R. and J.P. Habicht (1986). "Growth in early childhood in developing countries," in F. Falkner and J.M.Tanner (eds.), *Human Growth: A Comprehensive Treatise*, 2nd (ed.). New York and London: Plenum Press.

Martorell, R., U. Ramakrishnan, D.G. Schroeder, P. Melgar and L. Neufeld (1998). "Intrauterine growth retardation, body size, body composition and physical performance in adolescence", *European Journal of Clinical Nutrition* 52(1): S43-53.

Mason, J.B., M. Lotfi, N. Dalmiya, K. Sethuraman and M. Deitchler (2001). *The Micronutrient Report: Current Progress and Trends in the Control of Vitamin A, Iodine and Iron Deficiencies* (The Micronutrient Initiative).

Maxwell, D., Carol E. Levin, Margaret Armar-Klemesu, Marie T. Ruel, Soul Sutkover Morius and Clement Ahiadeke (2000). "Urban livelihoods and food and nutrition security in Greater Accra, Ghana", *Research Report 112*. Washington DC: International Food Policy Research Institute.

McGuire, J.B. and B.M. Popkin (1989). *Increasing Women's Resources for Nutrition in Developing Countries*. New York: 15th session of the ACC/SCN.

———. (1990). "Helping women improve nutrition in the developing world", *World Bank Technical Paper* No. 114. Washington DC: World Bank.

McJunkin, F.E. (1982). *Water and Human Health (USAID)*. Washington DC.

Meenakshi, J.V. (1996). "How important are changes in tastes? A state-level analysis of food demand", *Economic and Political Weekly* 31(50): 3265-269.

Meenakshi, J.V. and Ranjan Ray (1999). "Regional differences in India's food expenditure systems approach", *Journal of International Development* 11: 47-74.

Meenakshi, J.V., R. Ray and S. Gupta (2000). "Estimates of poverty for SC, ST and female-headed households", *Economic and Political Weekly* 35(31): 2748-754.

Meenakshi, J.V. and B. Vishwanathan (2001). "Developing country nutrition does improve with income: A look at calorie and protein intakes, 1983 to 1993-94", *Sarvekshana* 10-47. October–March.

———. (2003). "Calorie deprivation in rural India, 1983 – 1999/2000", *Economic and Political Weekly* 38(4): 369-75.

Melville, B., M. Williams, V. Francis, O. Lawrence and L. Collins (1988). "Determinants of childhood malnutrition in Jamaica", *Food and Nutrition Bulletin* 10(1): 43-7.

Micozzi, M.S., D. Albanes, D. Y.Jones and W.C. Chumlea (1986). "Correlation of body mass indices with weight, stature, and body composition in men and women in NHANES I and II ", *American Journal of Clinical Nutrition* 44: 725-31.

Miller, J.E. and S. Korenman (1994). "Poverty and children's nutritional status in the United States", *American Journal of Epidemiology* 140(3): 233-43.

Minhas, B.S. (1991). "On estimating the inadequacy of energy intakes: Revealed food consumption behaviour versus nutritional norms", *Journal of Development Studies* 28(1): 1-38.

Mishra, V.K., S. Lahiri and N.Y. Luther (1999). "Child nutrition in India", *National Family Health Survey Subject Reports* No. 14. Honolulu: East-West Center: IIPS.

Monsen, E.R., L. Hallberg, M. Layrisse, D.M. Hegsted, J.D. Cook, W. Mertz and C.A. Finch (1978). "Estimation of available dietary iron", *American Journal of Clinical Nutrition* 31: 134-41.

Mora, J. (1984). "Anthropometry in Prevalence Studies", in J. Brosek and B. Schurch (eds.), *Malnutrition and Behaviour: Critical Assessment of Key Issues* (Lausanne Nestle Foundation).

Mosley, W.H. and L.C. Chen (1984). "An analytical framework for the study of child survival in developing countries", *Population and Development Review* 10: 25-45.

Murphy, S.P., S.I. Barr and M.I. Poos (2002). "Using the new dietary reference intakes to assess diets: A map to the Maze", *Nutrition Reviews* 60(9): 267–75.

Murty, K.N. and R. Radhakrishna (1981). "Agricultural prices, income distribution and demand patterns in a low-income country", in Robert E. Kalman and J. Martinez (eds.), *Computer Applications in Food Production and Agricultural Engineering*. North-Holland Publishing Company.

Mwanri, L., A. Worsley, P. Ryan and J. Masika (2000). "Supplemental vitamin A improves anemia and growth in anemic school children in Tanzania", *Journal of Nutrition* 130: 2691-696.

NFHS-2 (1998-99). *National Family Health Survey Reports.* Mumbai, India: International Institute for Population Sciences.

National Nutrition Monitoring Bureau (1996). *Nutritional Status of Rural Population: Report of NNMB Surveys*. Hyderabad: National Institute of Nutrition, ICMR.

———. (2002). *Nutritional Status of Rural Population: Report of NNMB Surveys*. Hyderabad: National Institute of Nutrition, ICMR.

National Sample Survey (1983). *Thirty-Eighth Round*, Report No. 356. New Delhi: Department of Statistics.

———. (1999-2000). *Level and Pattern of Consumer Expenditure in India*, Report No. 457. New Delhi: Ministry of Statistics and Programme Implementation.

———. (1999-2000). *Employment and Unemployment Situation in India*, Report No. 458, vol. I. New Delhi: Ministry of Statistics and Programme Implementation.

———. (1999-2000). *Nutritional Intake in India 1999-2000*, Report No. 471. New Delhi: Ministry of Statistics and Programme Implementation.

———. (2000-01). *Household Consumer Expenditure and Employment-Unemployment Situation in India*, Report No. 476.

———. (2001-02). *Household Consumer Expenditure and Employment-Unemployment Situation in India*, Report No. 481.

Nutrition Foundation of India Bulletin (2004). *The Nutrition Scene in India: Time Trends* 25(2).

Olaniyan, O. (2002). "The effects of household resources and community factors on child health: Evidence from Nigeria", Paper prepared for presentation at the CSAE conference on *Understanding Poverty and Growth in Sub-Saharan Africa*, held at St Catharine's College. Oxford March 18-19.

OMNI Micronutrient Fact Sheets (1996): India. *http:///www.jsi.com/intl/omni/indi_pub.html*

Onyango, A., K.G. Koski and K.L. Tucker (1998). "Food diversity versus breastfeeding choice in determining anthropometric status in rural Kenyan toddlers", *International Journal of Epidemiology* 27(3): 484-89.

Opportunities for Micronutrient Interventions Project (OMNI) (1996). *Micronutrient Fact Sheet*, India.

Palmer-Jones, Richard and Kunal Sen (2001). "On India's poverty puzzles and statistics of poverty", *Economic and Political Weekly* 36(3): 211-17.

Park, K. (1997). *Park's Textbook of Preventive and Social Medicine*. Banarsidas Bhanot Publishers. Fifteenth Edition.

Payne, P. (1992). "Assessing Undernutrition: The need for a reconceptualization", in S.R. Osmani (eds.), *Nutrition and Poverty* WIDER Studies in Development Economics. Oxford University Press. pp.121-64.

Payne, P.R. (1975). "Safe protein-calorie ratios in diets. The relative importance of protein and energy intake as causal factors in malnutrition", *American Journal of Clinical Nutrition* 28: 281-86.

Payne, P. and M. Lipton (1994). "How third world rural households adapt to dietary energy stress: The evidence and the issues", *Food Policy Review* 2. Washington DC: International Food Policy Research Institute.

Peabody J., P. Gertler and A. Leibowitz (1998). "The impact of prenatal care quality on birth outcomes in Jamaica", *Health Policy* 43: 1-13.

Pitt, M.M. (1983). "Food preferences and nutrition in rural Bangladesh", *Review of Economics and Statistics* 65: 105-14.

Pitt, M.M. and M.R. Rosenzweig (1985). "Health and nutrient consumption across and within Farm Households", *Review of Economics and Statistics* 67(2): 212-22.

Planning Commission (2000). *Report of the Steering Committee of Nutrition*. New Delhi: Government of India.

Quisumbing, A. and J. Maluccio (2003). "Resources at marriage and intrahousehold allocation: Evidence from Bangladesh, Ethiopia, Indonesia, and South Africa", *Oxford Bulletin of Economies and Statistics* 65(3): 283–328.

Radhakrishna, R. and C. Ravi (1992). "Effects of growth, relative price and preferences on food and nutrition", *Indian Economic Review* 27: 303-23.

Ramakrishnan U., N. Aburto, G. McCabe and R. Martorell (2004). "Multimicronutrient interventions but not vitamin A or iron interventions alone improve child growth: Results of 3 meta-analyses", *Journal of Nutrition* 134(10): 2592-602.

Ramalingaswami, V., U. Jonsson and J. Rohde (1996). *Commentary: The Asian Enigma in the Progress of Nations*. New York: United Nations Children's Fund.

Rao C.H.H. (2000). "Declining demand for foodgrains in rural India: Census and implications", *Economic and Political Weekly* 35.

Rao C.R. (1973). *Linear Statistical Inference and its Applications*. New York: Wiley and Sons.

Ravallion, M. (1990). "Income effects on undernutrition", *Economic Development and Cultural Change* 38(3): 489-515.

Ricci J.A. and S. Becker (1996). "Risk factors for wasting and stunting among children in Metro Cebu, Philippines", *American Journal of Clinical Nutrition* 63: 966-75.

Rivera J.A., C. Hotz, T. Gonzalez-Cossio, L. Neufeld and A. Garcia-Guerra (2003). "The effect of micronutrient deficiencies on child growth: A review of results from community-based supplementation trials", *Journal of Nutrition* 133(11): 4010S–4020S.

Roy, Nilanjana (1996). "Series estimation of income elasticity of calorie intake across income classes", *Journal of Quantitative Economics* 12: 77–84.

———. (2001). "A semiparametric analysis of calorie response to income change across income groups and gender", *Journal of International Trade and Economic Development* 10: 93-109.

Ruel, Marie T. (2002). "Is dietary diversity an indicator of food security or dietary quality? A review of measurement issues and research needs", *Food Consumption and Nutrition Division Discussion Paper* No. 140, Washington DC: International Food Policy Research Institute.

———. (2003). "Operationalizing dietary diversity: a review of measurement issues and research priorities", *Journal of Nutrition Supplement* 133(11): 3911S-3926S.

Ruel, Marie T., James S. Garrett, Saul S. Morris, Daniel Maxwell, Arne Oshaug, Patrice Engle, Purnima Menon, Alisa Slack and Lawrence Haddad (1998). "Urban challenges to food and nutrition security: A review of food security, health, and care-giving in the cities", *Food Consumption and Nutrition Division Discussion Paper 51*. Washington DC: International Food Policy Research Institute.

Ryan, J.G., P.D. Bidinger, N.P. Rao, P. Pushpamma (1984). "The determinants of individual diets and nutritional status in six villages of southern India", *Research Bulletin no.* 7. Patancheru, Andhra Pradesh, India: International Crops Research Institute of the Semi-arid Tropics.

Sahn, D. (1990). "Malnutrition in Cote d'Ivoire: Prevalence and determinants", *Social Dimensions of Adjustment Working Paper* No. 4. World Bank.

Samson, T. and G. Lakech (2000). "Malnutrition and enteric parasites among under five children in Aynalem village, Tigray", *Ethiopian Journal of Health Development* 14(1): 67-75.

Schultink, W. and W. Gross (1996). "The influence of vitamin A on iron status and possible consequences for micronutrient deficiency alleviation programs", Proceedings of the workshop on *Micronutrient Interactions: Impact on Child Health and Nutrition*. Washington DC: International Life Sciences Institute Press.

Schultz, T.P. (1984). "Studying the impact of household economic and community variables on child mortality", *Population and Development Review* 10: 215-35.

Scrimshaw, N.S. and B.A. Underwood (1980). "Timely and appropriate complementary feeding of the breastfed infant: An overview", *Food Nutrition Bulletin* 2(2): 19-22.

Scrimshaw, N.S., C.E. Taylor and J.E. Gordon (1959). "Interaction of nutrition and infection", *American Journal of Medical Science* 237: 367-403.

Seckler, D. (1982). "Small but healthy: A basic hypothesis in the theory, measurement and policy of malnutrition", in P.V. Sukhatme (eds.), *Newer Concepts in Nutrition and their Implications for Policy*. Pune: Maharashtra Association for the Cultivation of Science.

Sen, A. (2000). "Estimates of consumer expenditure and its distribution: statistical priorities after NSS 55th round", *Economic and Political Weekly* 35(51): 4499-518.

Shah, C.H. (1983). "Food preference, poverty and the nutrition gap", *Economic Development and Cultural Change* 32: 121-148.

Shariff, A. and A.C. Mallick (1999). "Dynamics of food intake and nutrition by expenditure class in India", *Economic and Political Weekly* 34 (27): 1790-800.

Skoufias, E. (2001). "Is the calorie income elasticity sensitive to prices changes? Evidence from Indonesia", *Food Consumption and Nutrition Division Discussion Paper 141*. Washington DC: International Food Policy Research Institute.

Smith, L. and L. Haddad (2000). "Explaining child malnutrition in developing countries: A cross-country analysis", *Research Report* 111. Washington DC: International Food Policy Research Institute.

Smith, L.C., U. Ramakrishnan, A. Ndiaye, L. Haddad and R. Martorell (2003). "The importance of women's status for child nutrition in developing countries", *Research Report* 131. Washington DC: International Food Policy Research Institute.

Srinivasan, T.N. (1981). "Malnutrition: Some measurement and policy issues", *Journal of Development Economics* 8: 3-19.

———. (1985). "Malnutrition in developing countries: The state of knowledge of the extent of its prevalence, its causes and its consequences", (*Mimeo*).

Stein, A.J., J.V. Meenakshi, M. Qaim, P. Nestel, H.P.S. Sachdev, Z.A. Bhutta (2005). "Health benefits of biofortification: An ex-ante analysis of iron-rich rice and wheat in India", Paper presented at the *AAEA Annual Meeting*. July 24-27. Providence, RI.

Stoltzfus, R.J., H.M. Chwaya, J.M. Tielsch, K.J. Schulze, M. Albonico and L. Svioli (1997). "Epidemiology of iron deficiency anemia in Zanzibari schoolchildren: The importance of hookworms", *American Journal of Clinical Nutrition* 65: 153-59.

Strauss, J. (1982). "Determinants of food consumption in rural Sierra Leone: Application of the quadratic expenditure system to the consumption-leisure component of a household-firm model", *Journal of Development Economics* 11: 327-54.

———. (1984). "Joint determination of food consumption and production in Rural Sierra Leone: Estimates of household-firm model", *Journal of Development Economics* 14: 77-103.

———. (1990). "Households, communities and preschool children's nutrition outcomes: Evidence from Rural Cote d'Ivoire", *Economic Development and Cultural Change* 38(2): 231-62.

Strauss, J. and D. Thomas (1990). "The shape of the calorie expenditure curve", *Economic Growth Centre Discussion Paper* No. 595. Yale University.

Strauss, J. and D. Thomas (1995). "Human resources: empirical modeling of household and family decisions", in J.R. Behrman and T.N. Srinivasan (eds.), *Handbook of Development Economics*, volume IIIA. 1883-2024. Amsterdam: North-Holland.

———. (1998). "Health, nutrition, and economic development", *Journal of Economic Literature* 36(2): 766-817.

Subramanian, A. (2001). "Are income-calorie elasticity's really high in developing countries? Some implications for nutrition and income", National Council of Applied Economic Research, Paper prepared for the Session 10 (poverty and Inequality) of the *IUSSP XXIVth General Population Conference*. Salvadore. Brazil. August 18-24.

Subramanian, S. and A. Deaton (1996). "The demand for food and calorie", *Journal of Political Economy* 104(1): 133-62.

Sukhatme, P.V. (1982). "Poverty and malnutrition" in P.V. Sukhatme (ed.), *Newer Concepts in Nutrition and Their Implications for Policy*. Pune: Maharashtra Association for the Cultivation of Science.

———. (1987). "Poverty and malnutrition", *Economic and Political Weekly* 15: 83-89.

Sukhatme, P.V. and S. Margen (1982). "Autoregulatory homestatic nature of energy balance", *American Journal of Clinical Nutrition* 35: 355-65.

Sundaram, K. and S.D. Tendulkar (2002). "Recent debates on data base for measurement of poverty in India: Some fresh evidence", Paper presented at the *Workshop on Poverty Monitoring and Evaluation*, jointly organised by the World Bank and Planning Commission. New Delhi. January 11-12.

———. (2003). "Poverty in India in the 1990s: Revised results for all-India and 15 major states for 1993-94", *Economic and Political Weekly* 38(46): 4865-872.

Suryanarayana, M.H. (1995). "Growth, poverty and level of living: hypothesis, methods and policies", *Journal of Indian School of Political Economy* 7(2): 203-65.

Svedberg, P. (2000). *Poverty and Undernutrition: Theory, Measurement, and Policy*. Paperback Edition. India: Oxford University Press.

Tarozzi, A. (2004). "Calculating comparable statistics from incomparable surveys, with an application to poverty in India", Paper presented at the *North East Universities Development Consortium Conference*. Montreal. October 2004. Available at *http://www.hec.ca/neudc2004/Programme2.html*.

Taylor, C., A.A. Kielmann, C. Desweemer, I.S. Uberoi, H.S. Takulia, C.G. Neumann, W. Blot, H. Shankar, S. Vohra, G. Subbulakshmi, R.S. Sarma, R.L. Parker, C. McCord, N. Masih, D. Laliberte, N.S. Kielmann, D.N. Kakar and A. Forman (1978). "The Narangwal experiment on interaction of nutrition and infections: Project design and effects upon growth", *Indian Journal of Medical Research* 68(suppl.): 1-20.

Thomas, D. (1997). "Incomes, expenditures, and health outcomes: Evidence on intrahousehold resource allocation", in L. Haddad, J. Hoddinott and H. Alderman, Baltimore, Md. (eds.), *Methods, Models, and Policy*. International Food Policy Research Institute and Johns Hopkins University Press.

Thomas, D. and J. Strauss (1992). "Prices, infrastructure, household characteristics and child height", *Journal of Development Economics* 39(2): 301-31.

Thomas, D., V. Lavy, and J. Strauss (1996). "Public policy and anthropometric outcomes in the Cote d'Ivoire", *Journal of Public Economics* 61: 155-92.

Timmer, C.P. and Alderman (1979). "Estimating consumption parameters for food policy analysis", *American Journal of Agricultural Economics* 61: 982-87.

Tomkins, A.M. and F. Watson (1989). "Malnutrition and infections: A review", *Nutrition Policy Discussion Paper* No. 5, ACC/SCN, State of the Art Series.

Tseng, M., H. Chakraborty, D.T. Robinson, M. Mendez and L. Kohlmeier (1997). "Adjustment of iron intake for dietary enhancers and inhibitors in population studies: Bioavailable iron in rural and urban residing Russian women and children", *Journal of Nutrition* 127: 1456-468.

Underwood, B. and L. Hofvander (1982). "Appropriate timing for complementary feeding of the breast-fed infant", *Acta Paediat. Scand. Supplement* 294: 6-32.

UNICEF (1990). "Strategy for improved nutrition of children and women in developing countries", *UNICEF Policy Review Paper*. New York.

———. (1993). *Child Malnutrition: Progress Towards the World Summit for Children Goal*. New York: UNICEF.

United Nations (1996). *Preparation and Use of Food-based Dietary Guidelines*. New York: UN.

Vandana, S. and U. Singh (2002). *Vitamin-A Deficiency, Green Solutions versus Golden*. New Delhi: Research Foundation for Science, Technology and Ecology

Visaria, P. (2000). *Poverty in India during 1994—98: Alternative Estimates*. New Delhi: Institute for Economic Growth.

Victora, C.G. and F.J. Vaughn (1985). "Land tenure patterns and child health in southern Brazil: The relationships between agriculture production, malnutrition and child mortality", *International Journal of Health Services* 15: 253-74.

Ward, J.O. and J.H. Sanders (1980). "Nutritional determinants and migration in the Brazilian northeast: A case study of rural and urban Ceara", *Economic Development and Cultural change* 29: 141-63.

Waterlow, J.C. (1984). "Current issues in nutritional assessment by anthropometry", in J. Brozek, B. Schürch (eds.). *Malnutrition and Behaviour: Critical Assessment of Key Issues*. Lausanne, Switzerland: Nestlé Foundation.

Waterlow, J.C. and A.M. Tomkins (1992). "Nutrition and infection", in J.C. Waterlow (ed.), *Protein Energy Malnutrition*. London: Edward Arnold. pp. 290-324.

WHO (1986). *Technical Report Series* No. 732.

———. (1995). "Physical status: The use and interpretation of anthropometry, Report of a World Health Organization Expert committee", *WHO Technical Report Series* 854. Geneva.

———. (1998). "Complementary feeding of young children in developing countries: a review of current scientific knowledge", *WHO/NUT/98.1*, Davis, Geneva: University of California.

———. (2000). "Turning the tide of malnutrition: responding to the challenge of the 21st century", *WHO/NHD*.007, Geneva: WHO.

———. (2004). "Water, sanitation and hygiene links to health, Facts and figures 2004", at *http://www.who.int/water_sanitation_health/en/factsfigures04.pdf*

WHO/FAO (1996). *Preparation and Use of Food-based Dietary Guidelines*. Geneva: Nutrition Programme, World Health Organization.

Wolfe, B.L. and J.R. Behrman (1982). "Determinants of child mortality, health and nutrition in a developing country", *Journal of Development Economics* 11: 163-94.

Wolfe, B.L. and J.R.Behrman (1983). "Is income overrated in determining adequate nutrition?", *Economic Development and Cultural Change* 31: 525-50.

———. (1984). "Determinants of women's health status and health-care utilization in a developing country: A latent variable approach", *Review of Economics and Statistics* 56: 696-793.

———. (1987a). "Women's schooling and children's health: Are the effects robust with adult sibling control for the women's childhood background?", *Journal of Health Economics* 6(3): 239-54, September, Elsevier.

World Bank (1980). *World Development Report*. Washington DC: World Bank.

———. (1994). *Enriching Lives: Overcoming Vitamin and Mineral Malnutrition in Developing Countries*. USA: Washington DC.

Yimer, G. (2000). "Malnutrition among children in southern Ethiopia: Levels and risk factor", *Journal of Health Development* 14(3): 283-92.